AF333346

Random Thoughts

A Nursing Home Journal

Wanda R. Schwind

VANTAGE PRESS
New York / Los Angeles / Chicago

*To the handicapped,
particularly those confined to a wheelchair,
who, for reasons beyond their control,
are forced to live in a nursing home.*

The following publishers have generously given permission to use quotations from copyrighted works: From "The Dead Horse Hill Climb," originally printed in the *Christian Science Monitor*, July 18, 1985. From *The Complete Cherubs*, by Rebecca McCann, copyright © 1932, 1960 by Crown Publishers, Inc. From "Osark Symphony Croaks Along," copyright © 1986 *St. Louis Post-Dispatch*.

FIRST EDITION

Published by Vantage Press, Inc.
516 West 34th Street, New York, New York 10001

Manufactured in the United States of America
ISBN: 0-533-08130-0

Library of Congress Catalog Card No.: 88-90391

Preface

I wonder what I should call this little book of future jottings: *A Nursing Home Journal, A Diary of Sorts, My Think Book,* or just *Random Thoughts?* I opt for *Random Thoughts* because it best describes the helter-skelter workings of my mind.

Foreword

By J. A. Baer II, a Former Employer

My first encounters with Mrs. Schwind were early in my career with the Stix, Baer and Fuller Department stores in St. Louis. By the time I met her, she had already become one of the outstanding jewelry buyers in America. Much of her success was due to her personal dedication to any job she was about to perform. Her curiosity was a plus in being a very creative merchant.

I remember being with her in a tiny Austrian village which housed many postwar jewelers. While she was writing an order, I discovered a barrel of plastic beads which could be put together to form a bracelet or a necklace and were in many colors. I showed them to her, and she became extremely excited; we ended up buying the entire barrel. Out of that barrel came a piece of costume jewelry called the *popit.* It became one of the biggest selling items in America. That is only one simple story. There were many others.

Later when I became the president and chief executive of Stix, Baer and Fuller, I appointed Mrs. Schwind as our first woman merchandise manager. After she had proven herself as an outstandingly successful merchandising woman, we appointed her as the first woman vice president of our store. Over the years working with her was always a learning experience and an adventure.

When she retired, she and her loving husband, Morgan, settled down to a more quiet life. It wasn't long before she lost Morgan. A few months later she had a severe stroke.

Talking to her shortly afterwards, I told her I was sending her a gift—a tape recorder, so that she could write her memoires. Whether she did that or not, I don't know, but after putting herself into a retirement nursing home, she began writing about that home and the people in it.

She always said, "I can be as miserable as I let myself be." She decided that the challenge of writing this book would change her feeling of misery to one of accomplishment and happiness. She has always been a woman of accomplishment and as you read this book, you will understand why.

By Mrs Catherine J. Bono, a Nursing Home Administrator

I have been privileged in my life to have had many wonderful people pass my way. I have had many honors because I have been in a position of service to these people. None has ever moved me as much as being asked to contribute to the foreword of this book.

I have personally known Wanda for almost nine years, the length of time she has been living in a nursing home. I shared her experiences there as I watched her adjustment and acceptance of nursing home life. However, I feel as though I've known Wanda a lifetime since her journal, which covers two of these nine years, contains not only her thoughts and feelings, but her reminiscences as well. Thus I was given insight into the eighty years before the nursing home. These were the years that shaped the lady whose journal you are about to read.

Sometimes you will laugh, sometimes you will cry, always, as you read on, you will love. You will feel the empathy, the insight, the articulate, wonderful mind of the lady, and in the end you will love the gift she is giving to you, the reader. That gift is an education in growing older . . . accepting life.

By Mildred "Mickie" Fuller, a Fellow Nursing Home Resident

I met Wanda the first day I entered the nursing center. I remember feeling scared and alone. She offered me friendship, warm and instant. She granted me the excitement and adventure of a new friend. Her wit, enthusiasm, and compassionate consideration made my transition into a nursing center palatable.

As Wanda wrote this journal, she shared excerpts with me. I was fascinated. Her thoughts from the past link the present with insights to the future. She showed me strengths within myself and helped me to grow and to feel worthwhile. This special person added depth and dimension to my life. I believe that persons with and without disabilities will find equal reason for reading this book. They will both gain from her vision and ability to portray her feelings to others.

I admire her for publishing this candid journal, for her risk and hard work in living a wonderful full life. It is with honor and privilege that I applaud her work. Bravo, Wanda.

Christmas 1984

December 17

Today I am emotionally bankrupt. I think I am exhausted from pulling myself up by the boot straps—particularly since I've pulled so often, all or most of the elasticity has gone from the straps.

No matter what the next few days bring, today I'm going home for Christmas—if only in memory.

I want to remember Christmas 1977, my last Christmas with Morgan.

We were stretched out on the floor in front of the huge stone fireplace at Echo Valley, watching the embers burn low. We were holding hands and musing over the highlights of forty years of happy marriage. We also were dreaming dreams of the future. Our four-legged little people, Charlie, Mike, and Peppi, were stretched out alongside us, soaking up our warmth and happiness.

Just writing the above and reliving those happy hours helps to erase some of the real and imagined hurts and frustrations that engulf me here at Clayton on the Green from time to time—today especially!

Christmas Eve, December 24, 1984

Emily and Zane just left. I had ordered a bottle of champagne, and we spent the evening talking about computers, of all things.

Emily gave me a small crystal rabbit—a companion piece to the turtle that Cubby brought me from London a couple of years ago. Both are of Swarovski crystal. I can't help thinking "The Tortoise and the Hare" in crystal. What a lovely way to preserve a legend—and how both miniature crystals will look alongside the Swarovski paperweight (with the embedded Hapsburg coat of arms) that Eve and Ken recently brought to me from Vienna.

December 31, 1984

New Year's Eve—and time I start climbing to my mountaintop. From that pinnacle I can look back on the past year and continue making plans for 1985.

All in all, this has been a very happy holiday season—which is closing out a year that has been rich and fulfilling from a growing and spiritual standpoint. I no longer expect the peaks of happiness and ecstasy I once knew with Morgan. Instead, a warm contentment now enfolds me in a comforting embrace.

I've always put a high value on friendship, but this holiday season brought many of those friendships to full flowering. The phone calls, written messages, and personal visits touched me deeply because, I believe I've not only grown older and mellower in years, but I've grown in perception and appreciation.

January 1, 1985

Today is Morgan's birthday and my opportunity to make each day of the coming year a tribute to him by trying to make others as happy as he made me.

Tomorrow I start making new memories.

January 2, 1985

Not many new memories were made today, but I did relive some very pleasant old ones.

Tonight I listened to the Vienna Philharmonic, and what a montage of happy sights, hours, and friendships the music has painted for me—the Danube, the old opera house, Demels, the Vienna woods, the Sacher, four-power-rule, the magnificent Lippizaners, the Boys' Choir, Saint Stephen's. The list goes on and on. I believe Vienna will always be one of my favorite cities.

January 3, 1985

Writing in this book—or writing in or on anything—for me is an exercise in frustration. Holding the pen, paper, book, or whatever in one hand and trying to write with the same hand while the paper and/or et cetera skids all over the desk surface has me talking to myself.

Although I'm muttering to myself right now, I nevertheless want to jot down the fact that I listened to and thoroughly enjoyed Leontyne Price's *Aida* this evening. The music is still going around in my head and easing my frustration.

January 6, 1985

Sally Unger and Mary Halloway spent a couple of hours with me this afternoon. How pleasant it was to reminisce—to discuss books and our attitudes toward current world happenings. I realize again after a visit like this how much I appreciate stimulating conversation.

Shortly after their departure, the door of my room slowly opened and one of our wandering ladies peeked in—then gently closed the door. (This happens several times a day.) A bit spooky at times and in the words of one of the nurse's aides in reference to such goings-on "It must be a poultrygeist." I find that worth a hearty chuckle and a malaprop to end most malaprops.

January 14, 1985

Watching a segment of "Jewel in the Crown" on PBS last evening reminded me of two of the experiences I had in India during my first trip there in 1961.

I was en route to Bombay from Hong Kong and had to change planes in Calcutta (which may not have been the Black Hole then but was certainly, in my opinion, brown around the edges).

I had boarded the Air India plane and was huddled in the corner of my seat, observing the while that I was the only woman on the plane and the only person in Western dress. We were hardly more than airborne when the Indian steward, a Sikh, stopped in the aisle, alongside my seat, and making the traditional Indian sign of greeting said, "Bonne Marre," accompanied by the steeple-positioned fingers and bowed head. "You are a guest in my country. Is there anything I can do for you? Would you care for a cup of tea?"

Not too long after that, two other Indian gentlemen stopped by my seat and in essence said the same thing. One gentleman introduced himself as a professor at Bombay University. The other was an executive with Assam Oil Company. When we landed at Nangpur for a brief stopover, the two gentlemen invited me to join them for a cup of tea in the small Nangpur airport. I accepted, spent an enjoyable fifteen minutes, and have thought many times since how many Americans (generous and kind-hearted as we are) would take the trouble to say to a bewildered foreigner, "You are a guest in my country. Is there anything I can do to make your stay more pleasant?"

The other incident that left an indelible impression took place at Agra after I had admired my way through the Taj Mahal. As I walked along the fountainway leading from the entrance steps to the building, a small Indian boy approached me and wanted to know if he could be my guide around the grounds. "Only one rupee, lady." Of course, I accepted and as we approached the river alongside of which the Taj is built, I noticed several large black buzzards circling and quarreling overhead. At intervals, one or two of the birds would break away from the others and make a dive to the water. When I asked the Indian lad what was happening with the screaming birds, his reply was, "Guess somebody doesn't want a baby girl and has thrown it in the river."

January 15, 1985

I was late in getting around to reading *Megatrends*, but I find myself rethinking some of John Naisbitt's comments. At odd times of the day, I recall a couple of his observations, such as: "We are drowning in information and starving for knowledge." Another: "America's growth has gone through three stages—from farmer to laborer to clerk. The next step will be technician. But how will we fill the skilled jobs necessary to handle the new technology? There will be a labor shortage because our young men and women can't do simple arithmetic or write or read, let alone understand basic English."

In my opinion, *Megatrends* should be required reading for:

1. Young parents with school-age kids.
2. Literate young adults seeking direction.
3. Any oldster not too decrepit or foggy to learn.
4. All Americans who want to see our country regain its leadership in the world economy.

January 18, 1985

Sometimes I wonder what makes me tick, what are the components that make up the *me* that others perceive—or maybe it's the *me* of which only I am aware. I would guess those components would necessarily include:

1. My physical condition, which all in all is quite good. Of course, I'm paralyzed—but only on my left side! When I look around and see so many others worse off, I can't see where I have much right to complain.
2. My emotional state, which usually is pretty well balanced.
3. My mental attitude, which most of the time I can control by deliberate change of thought direction.
4. Environmental influence—both human and physical. When the human environment gets to me (as it does at times), I remind myself that there but for the grace of God go I. My physical environment is as pleasant as I can make it.
5. My faith, which is deep and abundant. Whenever the tears are close to the surface or whenever the lump in my throat is hard to swallow, I know if I turn my problems over to *Him,* my faith will soon lift me over the rough spots. It always has and it always will. The verse below helps:

Wings
by Earlyne Wheeler

Put wings on your attitude;
    Let your thoughts soar
Outward and upward
    Ground them no more.
Discard excess baggage of "ifs,"
    "buts," and "noes";
Send them away with the
    wind as it blows.
Cut through the darkness of delusion
    and doubt;
Turn the light high both
    within and without;
Rise above fog that limits
    your mind;
Keep moving upward 'til
    clear skies you find.
Stay on your course once
    you've risen above;
Maintain your position
    with wisdom and love.
Let wings on your attitude
    carry you through,
And blessings will follow
    in all that you do!

January 19, 1985
    I believe it was Ogden Nash who said,

When you're wrong, *admit it.*
When you're right, *shut up.*

With the above in mind, I'll write a note of apology to a friend regarding an erroneous statement I recently made and defended. And even if I'm right about the other points in our conversation, I'll make it a point to keep my big mouth shut.

Same day—but later

On a scale of one to ten, today has been a ten day.

January 20, 1985

I've been thinking about this one-to-ten day scale and how I started using it. It all began after I read an item in some paper or magazine. That item made a deep impression on me. Paraphrasing it, I believe I can make its underlying meaning come through:

It was 9:00 A.M. on a rainy, dreary Monday morning, and the elevator was filled with sour-faced office workers. As the elevator started to rise, the operator began humming a gay little tune and jiggling his feet.

One of the unsmiling passengers remarked, "Well, you certainly seem happy."

The pleasant reply was, "Yes, sir, I am! You see, I ain't never lived this day before!"

January 20, 1985

I watched President Reagan take the oath of office for his second term today. During the simple, eloquent ceremony, I couldn't help thinking how proud I am to be an American and how proud I am to have as a president a man who believes it isn't how much government can give the American people, but a president who has the faith to know how much the American people can do for themselves. (Oh dear, I'm afraid that paragraph exposes my political bent—as if my friends didn't know.)

Later

While waiting for the Super Bowl game to begin, I began to wonder just *why* I was so anxious for the 49'ers to win. I certainly didn't know enough of the fine points of football to know whether or not they were the better team, et cetera. I finally decided it all stemmed back to the fact that Morgan and I had always enjoyed San Francisco so much. Whether we were stopping at the Fairmont, meeting friends at the Top of the Mark, or just strolling through Fisherman's Wharf, the name of that old town always brings pleasant memories. What a sentimental old lady I am!

January 21, 1985

The second swearing-in ceremony for Ronald Reagan took place today, and I watched every minute of it from invocation to benediction. I listened intently to Mr. Reagan's inaugural address and thought it moving, forward-looking, reassuring, and completely within the confines of common sense. All through the address, I kept thinking how great it is to be an American and how happy I was that I had voted for him both in '80 and in '84 and would again if it were possible for him to seek another term.

In my opinion, the Reagan administration has turned the direction of the country around to where basic values and traditions are once more meaningful.

And I certainly don't think having a love affair with our country is something of which to be ashamed.

January 23, 1985

Whenever I feel pressured and confined to a restricted life, I try to remember what pressure and environment do to carbon. Carbon is that nonmetallic element especially found in organic substances. Whether carbon turns into the graphite used in lead pencils or into brilliant crystalline formations called diamonds depends almost entirely upon the circumstance or environment in which the element is found and the pressure that it has withstood. Both diamond and graphite are almost pure carbon.

Naturally, I prefer that my outlook take on a diamond quality rather than the leaden look of graphite. Between the two extremes are coal and marcasite, both of which contain a preponderance of carbon. Coal is utilitarian; marcasite is ornamental and, when faceted and polished, is attractively used in fashion jewelry.

January 25, 1985

I'll call them Annie and Joe. Actually, they are two residents who live here at the nursing home. She is seventy-nine, tiny, birdlike, and feisty. He is eighty, stubborn and pugnacious. Both have a talent for bickering and making the other angry.

I don't know what triggered this particular outburst, but Annie must have said something that made Joe furious. He was standing in the middle of a corridor shaking his forefinger at Annie. In obvious rage, he said, "You go to hell!"

Annie, shaking her forefinger just as vehemently, replied, "You can run your own errands!"

January 26, 1985

I found myself thinking critically of just about everything this morning. I thought the breakfast table sloppily set, my table-mates complaining, the sun blinding as it streamed through the east windows of the dining room, *and* to top it all off, my foot hurt, all because the evening nurse had failed to put on my foot the plastic cast that I wear while sleeping to position, support, and train the damaged muscles and tendons.

Finally it has dawned upon me that my criticism of others is but a reflection of some or even the same fault in me—namely: self-interest, negligence, thoughtlessness, or just plain carelessness. Those qualities I certainly exercise at times.

It was only yesterday that I failed to have my thirsty plants watered. And this morning I was mentally blaming everyone else for not having remembered.

Too, it has been almost a week since I promised that sweet third-grader (my pen pal) that I'd answer her letter immediately. As soon as I finish struggling with this recalcitrant page, I'll write to her.

*   *   *

We go through three stages of growth in our lifetime. Those stages are: youth, middle age, and "My, how good you look!" To qualify for the last, one must be my vintage. Whenever anyone says to me, "My, how good you look," my first impulse is to giggle. Then I smile, "pleased as punch" that my age has been recognized so pleasantly.

*   *   *

Jim sat with folded hands, waiting—waiting for Jim Jr. to pick him up and take him for that promised visit home. The promise had been made two months ago when Jim had been brought to the nursing center. Jim knew that his son was busy and had a life of his own to live. That knowledge, however, didn't make the waiting any easier.

*   *   *

Retreating within oneself usually takes one of two directions:

1. Communing with and seeking guidance from that still, small voice that exists within each one of us.
2. Tapping the self-feeding ego of self-interest. That too abounds in each of us.

Sometimes at night loneliness creeps in on Sandburg's little cat feet, filling every nook and cranny of the body with a heaviness that hurts.

I think the aching teenager and the forgotten old feel that loneliness most. Suicide too often has become the way out for the young. The old philosophically look forward to death as a release.

*   *   *

To this day, I remember the illustration my father used in teaching me religious tolerance. I was a young girl but old enough to know the meaning of and to visualize a wheel.

My father asked if I knew what a wheel was.

I answered, "Yes."

He then asked if I knew what a hub was.

I recall saying, "Yes, it's that thing in the middle."

His reply was, "Yes, and 'that thing' is the core or center of what I'm about to tell you."

He then asked if I knew what the spokes and rim were. I knew about the spokes, but was a bit hazy about the rim.

He replied that when he was finished talking with me, I'd understand about the rim. He continued, saying I'd meet and know many people during my lifetime. Many would remain just acquaintances, some would become fast friends, and there would be others with whom I'd disagree. If that disagreement was over religion, he'd like for me to remember the wheel. He then said if that person with whom I disagreed believed that there was a power greater than he or any human being, then his hub would become his goal of religious understanding.

He said I'd probably call my goal "God," because that was what I had been taught. Others might call it "spirit" or "principle." Still others might call it "soul." A scientist might call it "energy." No

10

matter the name as long as he believed in a universal power greater than man.

The spokes, my father said, were the pathways by which each person traveled to reach his goal. One spoke might be Catholicism, another Judaism or Buddhism or some branch of Protestantism, et cetera.

My father's admonition was, "Don't ever, as long as you live, criticize anyone for traveling a different spoke than you. That person is probably as serious and trying as hard as you to reach and understand his hub."

By that time, I was getting curious about the rim and asked what the rim had to do with hub and spokes.

My father's reply was, "That's the faith that holds everything together. Make certain your faith or rim is always strong."

January 30, 1985

I've thought all day it was time I started making plans for a new start (my sixth) in learning to walk better and to try again to lead a less restricted life.

Prior to this, I have made five other new beginnings: They were:

1. When following my stroke (six years ago) I first learned how to take steps wearing a steel brace on my leg and using a quad cane.
2. When my left foot muscles reverted to the classic stroke position and accelerated and more concentrated therapy was required. It was then that I started wearing heavy surgical boots for daily therapy. My more feminine, soft "sitting-around" shoes will not support a steel brace, and I cannot stand without a brace.
3. When I broke my hip and had to start the learning process all over.
4. and 5. when following two tendon surgeries I found it necessary each time to start over again.

Now I want to get out of the surgical boots, which I still wear for daily therapy, and out of my wheelchair on occasion and into something that will permit me to look a little less like something out of "M*A*S*H*."

All I need for a fresh start now are:

1. A new pair of orthopedic oxfords.
2. A determined attitude (which I have).
3. As much effort as I can muster.

I believe, and with God willing, there will be no need for a seventh attempt.

*   *   *

Alice's curly white hair, twinkling blue eyes, and angelic smile belie her caustic tongue and frequent use of unexpected expletives. Her remarks are usually timely and humorous, often vitriolic, and to the point because they always contain an element of truth.

A new private duty nurse, a Miss Smith, a short, pleasant-faced woman with a beam wider than needed for symmetry, walked by Alice recently.

The latter blurted out, "Lady, for your height, you have the biggest butt I've ever seen."

Miss Smith stopped, looked at Alice for a split second, then laughingly said, "Grandma, now I know I'm going on that diet to-day!"

"Grandma," Alice spluttered. "You have a nerve!"

That exchange took place over a week ago, and Alice hasn't been heard making an unkind remark since.

February 1, 1985

There has been considerable comment lately in the press and on TV about the closing down, for health reasons, of one of the largest nursing homes in St. Louis.

Today, a family member of one of the residents here asked me if I was satisfied with the care I receive at COTG [Clayton-on-the-Green]. My answer was an unequivocal "yes."

Later, I made a mental list of what I thought comprises good nursing home care.

First and foremost, I believe, is a director or administrator who is *people-oriented.* One whose love for and care of the old, ill, and handicapped is genuine and expressed in action and not in grandstanding statements and preachments, which usually fool no one, least of all the old, ill, and handicapped. Families, I think, tend to believe what they want to believe.

When the director is motivated by real love and concern for others, then he or she soon becomes the role model for all others employed in the facility.

It is then that a humanistic or holistic (as I believe it's called today) approach is taken toward health care. All bases should be touched, not just physical care, but also giving attention to the emotional, mental, environmental, and spiritual well-being of the patient or resident.

From all I hear and read, I sincerely believe COTG does an above average job in total health care:

1. The facility is kept and maintained hygienically clean. This translates into knowledgeable and caring dietary, maintenance, housekeeping, and laundry staffs.
2. While not always to my particular taste, I know our meals are well balanced, carefully prepared, and nutritious.
3. An all-out effort is made to keep us active, happy, and entertained. Being in a wheelchair has not been a deterrent to my participation, thanks to the care and patience of the staff. Trips to the symphony, Muny Opera, "Pop" concerts, and theater are often on the activity agenda, as well as entertainment brought to the home. This includes movies, small bands, singing groups, and other entertainers. Too, there are cooking, quilt-making, and other craft classes. Also, supervised games such as Bingo, brain quizzes, and Trivial Pursuit. There is always something available to keep the residents interested.

Of course, there are things not to my liking:
Being a very private person, I believe the invasion of my privacy on occasion annoys me the most. I realize the nurses and aides are so accustomed to nudity and body functions they think nothing of barging into one's room or bath without knocking on the door. I dislike, too, the crude and sometimes even vulgar expressions that not too infrequently spice the conversations of some staff members. (I believe this isn't too uncommon in hospitals either.)

And I do become irked when the RNs and LPNs (not all) can't or won't do the work of an aide when It's necessary. The nurses frequently say, "Wait a minute; I'll call an aide. She'll transfer you" or "She'll help you with your shoe" or whatever.

And I haven't yet learned to like overcooked, mushy vegetables or greasy-skinned baked chicken.

It's quite obvious the pluses for COTG far overshadow the minuses. All of which reminds me of a story I heard years ago about an old small-town couple who were soon to celebrate their seventy-fifth wedding anniversary.

The young editor of the town weekly decided he'd personally interview the couple and make a front-page story of the upcoming celebration.

When interviewed, George, the husband, said that the marriage had been wonderful, that Martha had been a perfect wife, that he and Martha had known seventy-five years of marital bliss. His eulogizing went on and on.

Finally, the young editor (recently divorced) thought he'd better talk with Martha. Surely there had been at least a few arguments and disagreements, and she might be freer with her comments.

Turning to Martha, the editor said, "Martha, do you mean to tell me that in all these years, you never once thought of divorcing George?"

Her reply was, "Divorce George and spoil a good marriage? I should say *not,* young man, but I can't tell you the number of times I wanted to kill him."

February 2, 1985

I traveled to Italy, vicariously, all afternoon. I revisited the rolling hills and winding roads of Tuscany, Volterra, the alabaster "factories," and Volterra's Museo Guarnacci—all because the February issue of *Smithsonian* contains an intriguing article on the Etruscans, those people who once inhabited almost the whole of the Italian peninsula. No one really knows from where these people came or anything at all about their language. Yet their excavated artifacts and the remains of their engineering feats indicate they were a cultured, skilled, and civilized people when Rome was but a settlement of mud huts.

Herodotus first guessed the origin of the Etruscans, and scientists have been guessing ever since. The *Smithsonian* article says: "They seemingly burst full-blown onto the world stage about 800 to 750 B.C."

I first became interested in Etruscan lore when I visited Volterra to buy alabaster items for SBF. On one of my trips there in years past, I was buying in one of the "factories" when the owner (I believe his name was Bessie) after showing me the regular line of alabaster items brought out a copy of an Etruscan museum piece, made in alabastrite and colored black to resemble black Bucchero pottery.

That pottery had in turn been created by the Etruscans to resemble the metal they so skillfully worked. I didn't feel the replica was a salable item for a department store, so I didn't buy it for SBF, but I did buy it for myself. Upon my return home I found no enthusiasm for the Etruscans or the replica. Therefore, I didn't reconsider ordering the item for SBF

Imagine my surprise today when I turned to page 51 in the *Smithsonian* to find a picture of the original of my replica. The original was a "stylization of attenuated bronze youth, second century B.C."

My copy is only inexpensive black alabastrite, but it meant "Etruscan" to me.

Like so many other things I've looked for since my life-style changed and I sold my home and Echo Valley, I can't find it! However, I've had the enjoyment today of remembering, and I'm ever so grateful I was able to visit so many faraway places during my working years.

I never get bored because I have so much to remember and think about.

* * *

Lily was a new resident. She was eighty-three and neither acted nor looked her age. An aide complimented her upon her appearance and alertness, to which Lily pertly replied, "Humph! All these compliments just because I know my ass from my elbow."

* * *

The many-faceted in-depth article on the elderly in America in the last issue of *Wilson's Quarterly* is, in my opinion, well worth reading. The statistics are eye-opening and the observations by such writers and scholars as Albert Rosenfeld, Timothy James, and Andrew Achenbaum are very thought-provoking.

February 5, 1985

Growing older has never bothered me. In fact, I don't believe I've given it too much thought one way or the other, except on one occasion, not too long ago, when I convinced myself that I had been born too soon. Old-fashioned as it may sound, I found and still find myself at odds with the permissiveness of today's world. I find the almost cavalier acceptance of divorce, premarital sex, pornography, strident feminism, street crime, et cetera, et cetera, et cetera, extremely distasteful to me. The rejection of the aforementioned were and are values upon which my life has been structured.

I do believe, however, the pendulum is swinging back to the traditions that mean so much to many of us oldsters.

Speaking of age, I like to recall Karl Wilson Baker's comments on age.

> Let me grow lovely, growing old—
> So many fine things do;
> Laces, and ivory, and gold,
> And silks need not be new;
> And there is healing in old trees,
> And old streets a glamour hold;
> Why may not I, as well as these,
> Grow lovely, growing old.

* * *

If I were starting my schooling today, space study, I believe, would be an overriding interest—not to become an astronaut, but to become an astrophysicist.

I have never thought there was any conflict between science and religion. Actually, I believe one complements the other. And what would be more challenging than to study and exchange ideas with those questing people who are trying to find out

1. How our universe began.
2. Where our universe is going.
3. How our universe will end.

My pseudo-intellectual outburst above is occasioned by an article I just read about Alan Guth, an astrophysicist from M.I.T. who has come up with a revolutionary theory describing an "inflationary universe that has answered so many of the previous unsolvable problems about the early universe that it took the fields of cosmology, astrophysics and particle physics by storm."

I know enough to know that I really haven't the foggiest idea of what it's all about. But wouldn't it be fun to know?

*   *   *

I'm learning! Never ask an oldster how he or she feels (unless you really want to know and have an hour to spend). Why? Because he or she will tell you in microscopic detail. Be prepared to ask the right questions and make sympathetic comments such as: "Really, that long in intensive care?"; "and that was your third operation?"; "You even had a second opinion?"; or "And you were on the operating table four hours and thirty-seven minutes?" and include "Oh, dear!" and as many "My, my's" as you can squeeze in between his or her descriptive comments.

Unless you make the right responses, accompanied by an unbelieving look on your face, you'll be thought a dum-dum and/or an unsympathetic clod.

*   *   *

What self-serving, egotistical critters we humans are (and I am no exception). I'm thinking about what an old professor of mine often said: "Whenever you find yourself feeling smug about some good deed you've done, just remember you received more or at least as much pleasure from it as the recipient. Altruism is in the final analysis nothing but out-and-out egoism."

How very right that statement is. This morning I laboriously wheelchaired my way over a thick carpet to find an aide for a fellow resident who couldn't quite make it over the carpeting.

The resident was happy to get the assistance, but I found myself literally patting myself on the back for having been the Good Samaritan. I was beginning to feel smug. It was I-I-I.

I had exerted the necessary effort to seek help.

I had found the aide.

I had pleased the resident.

but

What was the warm glow inside me? Nothing in the world but self-pleasure (egoism) because I had given pleasure to another (altruism).

February 6, 1985

Listening to President Reagan's state-of-the-union address this evening, I couldn't help thinking how well he reflects the feelings of so many Americans. He touches our hearts because he says so eloquently what so many of us feel but don't know how to express in words.

As he spoke about hope, opportunity, free enterprise, and our future, Americanism welled up inside me as I'm sure it did in many others. I thought how apropos were Van Dyke's "America for Me" and Israel Zangwill's observations on what makes an American. Excerpts from each flashed through my mind, but it has been so long ago since I read them, I know I can't repeat or quote either now in its entirety. Tomorrow I'll try to find the full texts of each.

February 7, 1985

I located "America for Me" and Zangwill's comments in an anthology lent to me by Barbara Fick.

America For Me
by Henry Van Dyke

'Tis fine to see the old world
    and travel up and down
Among the famous palaces
    and cities of reknown,
To admire the crumbly castles
    and the statues of the Kings—

But now I think I've had enough
        of antiquated things.

So it's home again, home again,
        America for me!
My heart is turning home again
        and there I long to be
In the land of youth and freedom
        beyond the ocean bars,
Where the air is full of sunlight
        and the flag is full of stars.

Oh, London is a man's town, there's
        power in the air;
And Paris is a woman's town, with
        flowers in her hair;
And it's sweet to dream in Venice,
        and it's great to study Rome,
But when it comes to living, there
        is no place like home.

I like the German fir-woods, in
        green battalions drilled;
I like the gardens of Versailles with
        flashing fountains filled;
But, oh, to take your hand, my dear,
        and ramble for a day
In the friendly western woodland
        where nature has her way!

I know that Europe's wonderful
        yet something seems to lack
The past is too much with her and
        The people looking back.
But the glory of the present is to make
        the future free—
We love our land for what she is
        and what she is to be.

> Oh, it's home again, and home again,
>   America for me!
> I want a ship that's westward bound,
>   to plough the rolling sea,
> To the blessed land of Room Enough
>   beyond the ocean bars
> Where the air is full of sunlight
>   and the flag is full of stars.

Zangwill's comments were:

America is God's crucible, the great melting-pot where all the races of Europe are melting and reforming! Here you stand, good folk, think I when I see them at Ellis Island, here you stand in your fifty groups, with your fifty languages and histories, and your fifty blood hatreds and rivalries. But you won't be long like that, brothers, for these are the fires of God you've come to—these are the fires of God. A fig for your feuds and vendettas! Germans and Frenchmen, Irishmen and Englishmen, Jews and Russians—into the crucible with you all! God is making the American. The real American has not yet arrived. He is only in the crucible, I tell you—he will be the fusion of all races, the common superman.

*   *   *

"Count your blessings" is not an idle admonition. It was following the loss of my beloved Morgan, which was followed within the year by my having a severe stroke, that I started counting my blessings.

Having no family (brothers, sisters, parents, children, or immediate relatives) and being unable to care for myself, it was necessary that I move into a nursing home. All that I loved—my husband, home, my way of life—all had been swept away; my world had collapsed.

My adjustment from one life-style to another was very difficult. Counting and actually writing down my blessings did much to ease my hurting heart and help me to accept my new life.

I found a blank stenographic notebook and started listing every good thing I could think of that I had ever experienced. I was amazed at all the wonderful things that I had been taking for granted—simple things like the fragrance of freshly brewed coffee or spice cake baking in the oven, the availability of the morning paper, the sunshine that greeted me upon awakening, et cetera.

I recorded all the advantages I'd had as a child—my parents' love for me, the education they'd given me, their guidance, et cetera.

Before I knew it, I had filled one side of the notebook and had flipped the book over to fill the opposite pages. I had jotted down everything I could think of—from the strength given me by supportive friends, to my mother's delightful sense of humor and the love I always felt from animals, to how good I always felt after a whirlpool bath.

That practical exercise in writing down my blessings did a great deal in altering my attitude from a negative to a positive approach. I recommend it to anyone who is seeking a happier life.

Today my philosophy is: I can be as happy as I *want* to be, or I can be as miserable as I *let* myself be.

And I don't choose to be miserable. It only makes everyone else miserable, too, and it's such a waste of time and energy.

*   *   *

It's truly sad when memory fails and confusion sets in. It is then that the fine line between fantasy and reality is crossed, not only once, but criss-crossed many times.

I recently overheard the following conversation taking place between two attractive elderly ladies. They were standing in a corridor, debating whether they should go to the dining room—or to find the room that they shared.

The one woman, tall, regal in posture, said, "Let's go to our room. Do you think we can find it?"

The other woman, a bit shorter but equally stately, replied, "I don't know. Do you think the nurses hide it from us on purpose?"

The first lady replied, "That wouldn't be a very nice thing for them to do, would it? Let's ask that nurse over there. . . . Surely she'll help us."

With that they locked arms and started walking up the hall, seeking the room from which they'd just emerged.

February 9, 1985

Tonight I am having one of my "old-tyme" sinus flare-ups—the first I've had in ten years.

The postnasal drip has left my throat raw and so sore I can hardly swallow. This is accompanied by a throbbing headache and stomach queasiness.

But . . . a hot whirlpool, a couple of Tylenol, and I'll be as good as new—that is, unless I have to sit up most of the night in order to breathe, in which case I'll greet the morning bleary-eyed and bulbous-nosed.

Oh, the joys of sinusitis! No one ever dies of it. One just wants to!

February 10, 1985

This is going to be a ten day! I know!

It was off to a good start when Sue (one of our very competent, extremely likable aides) came into my room at seven this morning to plump my bed pillows and give me fresh water.

I asked her to explain to my tablemates at breakfast that I was breakfasting in my room only because I felt like pampering my sinus headache.

I asked that because about three years ago, one of our very talkative residents had me stricken with cancer—all because I had an upset stomach and couldn't face food for a couple of meals.

Sue, nodding understandingly, said, "Better than that, I'll just tell them it's the wrong time of the month for you."

With that, I cracked up, and I've been laughing ever since.

February 11, 1985

I looked across the crowded dining room this evening and thought we all wear masks of one kind or another. Some of us wear thoughtful masks, others smiling or bored ones. Each conceals our emotions and thoughts so well it is difficult for someone else to tell what we really feel or think. It is hard for others to know what heartache or loneliness lies hidden deep within.

I wondered about the gentleman at the next table. Was he angry, disgusted, or dyspeptic? The lady three tables over, was the hungry look on her face a longing for food or for love and affection? And her tablemate? That lady's mouth hadn't stopped moving. Was she eating or gossiping? From the pleased look on her face it could have been either.

I wonder if anyone has guessed what my mask conceals.

Later tonight, I knew I had lost my knack for hiding my feelings. I let my physical hurts override my understanding of others. Those hurts filled me with self-pity and resentment because others didn't understand my feelings.

I'm very ashamed of my selfish attitude and obvious resentment.

At my age and with my working experience, I should have expected and discounted the "buck passing" I heard all evening.

It was stupid of me to let myself get so upset. My throbbing foot and raw throat hurt less than the loss of my self-esteem for letting my emotions get out of control.

*　　*　　*

Methinks it's time to climb to my mountaintop. I've been too long in the valley. The climb is never very easy, but with each step forward the pathway becomes smoother. I know because I've trod it many times. From trial and error trudging. I've learned there are two pathways. The first one is of negative thinking and dwelling upon past mistakes. The second is one of thinking and climbing upward with expectation. By climbing and looking upward I'm not as tempted (as I have been on occasion) to jump off into oblivion.

How melodramatic that sounds. When I think back upon all that has transpired since my stroke, the above is less dramatic than the reality of what I tried to do a couple of times.

There were times at first when I was certain life wasn't worth living. There were times at the hospital when I even tried to maneuver my wheelchair into a position where I could open a stair door and accidentally roll down one of the stairways between floors.

During a Caribbean cruise I took shortly after coming to COTG, I spent most of my time trying to figure out how I could accidentally wheelchair into the water.

It's obvious none of my efforts came to fruition—and for that I am grateful!

Now that I have my head screwed on properly, I find that life is very much worth living and most days can become ten days if I but try.

February 16, 1985

I was asked today if I was as contented, happy, and satisfied with life as I pretended.

Pretended? That word brought me up short.

Am I pretending?

Am I actually contented and satisfied with life?

Am I actually happy? Or

Am I nothing but an aging Pollyanna?

The answer is yes to each question.

I am what I think because my thoughts reflect the me I want to be. And I believe that "want to be me" will eventually become the "real me."

I so firmly believe that if I want something enough and strive hard enough that something will become a reality.

I also believe the disappointments, setbacks, and heartaches along the way are but tests of my physical and spiritual strength and endurance.

I've found that with each obstacle I've overcome, the more I believe in my ability to accept life as it comes to me.

I've learned that with acceptance come serenity, contentment, peace of mind, and strengthened faith.

I sincerely believe I am what I think I am or, as some say, what I pretend I am.

February 17, 1985

After reading my last entry, I've concluded that an aging Pollyanna, like an inept do-gooder, is either an insufferable bore or an out-and-out pain in the neck.

To keep from becoming either a bore or a pain and to refrain from drowning in my own complacency, I'd better remind myself of a couple of my most obnoxious traits:

1. I'm opinionated.
2. I tend to be bossy.
3. Surprisingly, I'm overly sensitive.
4. I cry easily. A snuggly puppy, a beautiful sunset, a baby's smile, a moonlight garden—almost any lovely or tender thing can turn on the spigot.

5. Rightly or wrongly and sometimes stupidly, I'm always for the underdog.

February 20, 1985

Annie and Joe were at it again. She, flushed and angry, had just said, "If you were my husband, I'd give you poison."

Joe nonchalantly replied, "If you were my wife, I'd certainly take it."

(Lady Astor and Sir Winston couldn't have played the scene better.)

February 21, 1985, A.M.

Tonight is the "Friends" preview of Maori artifacts and tribal rituals (performed by Maori elders) at the St. Louis Art Museum.

I'd like so much to attend, but it's raining and as taking me any place in a wheelchair, even in good weather, is a major production, I just haven't the nerve to impose upon any of my friends by asking to be taken, et cetera.

St. Louis is one of the three cities in the U.S. to even show this collection. (The other two are New York and San Francisco.) As the tribal treasures (not the elders) will remain in St. Louis until May 26, I'll make an attempt to see them before the closing date.

February 21, 1985, P.M.

The passing years have taught me many things, things I thought I knew (but didn't) when I was young. Now I appreciate the value of time. How I squandered it in days gone by!

Making every minute and hour count never occurred to me when I was hurrying to "grow up" or rushing to accomplish something I thought important at the time.

Too, now I believe I know the meaning of love, but I wonder if one ever comprehends the miracles it can perform. No—I think not—not until that love has been taken from you.

And friendship? Courage? Loyalty? Integrity? All those sterling qualities I mouthed but did not appreciate or really know until their heartfelt warmth bolstered my everyday living.

There are so many truths to be realized by living each day to its fullest.

* * *

From John Naisbett's Megatrends

As we move from an industrial to an information society we will use our brain power to create instead of our physical power and the technology of the day will extend and enhance our mental ability.

Our most formidable challenge will be to train people to work in the information society. Jobs will become available, but who will possess the high tech skills to fill them? Not today's graduates who cannot manage simple arithmetic or write basic English and certainly not the unskilled unemployed drop-outs who cannot even find work in the old sunset industries.

Farmer, laborer, clerk and the next transition will be technician. But that is a major jump and will be in a skill level.

We are letting Japan and the "New Japans" of the Third World take over the lead in electronics, biotechnology and the other sunrise sectors.

We are flooded with information and starved for knowledge.

As Naisbett says, "What a fantastic time to be alive."

February 24, 1985

She was complaining bitterly about doctors in general and one in particular whom she blamed entirely for her "crippled condition."

Not knowing anything about the situation, I merely told her about two upbeat experiences I'd known:

When my husband, Morgan, was so very ill and I was told surgery was necessary, a Dr. Kenneth Bennett was recommended as the surgeon to perform the operation. I didn't know Dr. Bennett or anything about him, but I did inquire around and heard only glowing reports about his surgical skill and medical ability.

When I met Dr. Bennett for the first time, I said, "I've been told you are the very best in your field."

Instead of answering as so many doctors might have, saying there were other surgeons who were capable of performing the operation, et cetera, Dr. Bennett looked at me, no doubt sensing my utter despair and fear, and said matter-of-factly, "That's right; I am!" That single forthright declaration dispelled my fear and gave me the confidence I needed. I can say now I know Dr. Bennett's ability, both medical and psychological, prolonged Morgan's life by many weeks.

Within the year, following the loss of Morgan, I had a stroke, which I learned later was quite severe. While Dr. Bennett was not my doctor, he did stop by my hospital room on occasion to say "hello" and wish me well.

One day he said, "You know if what has happened to you in so short a time had happened to me, I think I'd be full of rage. I'm not sure I could handle it as well as you're handling it." That, coming from that wonderful young doctor, started me on my way uphill. I said to myself, "See here, old lady, you just better get up on your feet and start climbing." That was some six years ago. In the interim, Dr. Bennett has been made chief of staff of general surgery at Jewish Hospital, one of St. Louis's best hospitals.

About a month or so ago, the *St. Louis Post-Dispatch* carried a long article about Dr. Bennett and some of the skillfull and intricate surgery he performs.

I often pat myself on the back for being so perceptive about him back in 1978–79.

There have been times when I let annoying and disagreeable tasks become wearisome burdens. I recall twice in particular when I permitted those burdens to become heavy crosses that I carried grudgingly as I trudged along.

What I didn't see then as I do now is that if only I'd rolled up my sleeves and attacked those tasks head-on, they soon would have been small chores with little chance of becoming burdens and if only when I let those tasks become burdens I'd shifted their weight by changing my attitude, those burdens would never have become heavy crosses.

As for the crosses, they were never as heavy as I'd let myself imagine. I've learned the hard way that God never put on my shoulders more than I could carry.

Now *if only* I'll remember all the *if only* alternatives I should have chosen and do something about *if onlys* that are sure to come up in the days ahead. If only I'll use that lump between my ears and think things through.

February 26, 1985

At the moment I'd like to "lay back my ears and bray" or pound my desk with the shoe that has been left in the middle of the floor (beyond my reach).

Instead of either childish temper tantrum, I'll write out my frustrations. I've found that to be good therapy.

My day started off with a breakfast that was a disaster. Threading my wheelchair way between tables that had been placed too close together in the dining room, I arrived at my table to find that glasses of fruit juice and water had been carelessly, sloppily set on the place mats. Water was dripping off the side of the table. I didn't see the fruit juice until the sleeve of a new sweater I was wearing had mopped up most of it. However, it wasn't until the poached egg I was served not only appeared to be but was, for all practical purposes, uncooked. It wasn't until then that I felt like stalking (as if one could stalk in a wheelchair) out of the dining room in outraged womanhood. Instead, I ate a bowl of cereal, all the while using my napkin to soak up the juice on my sticky sleeve. I felt somewhat better by the time I arrived back in my room—only to find that a new aide had left one of my bedroom slippers in the middle of the floor and the other on top of a chest of drawers.

Compared to what is happening in the world today, nothing that occurred this morning is of much consequence. It only upset my little world—and made me as waspish as one of those swatted-at angry insects.

A little better supervision in the dining room and use of a little judgment by the young dietary staff would smooth away many ruffled feelings at mealtime.

Referring to judgment, that, unfortunately, is something that can't be taught. One acquires that only by day-to-day living and experience and by one's ability to learn and grow in perceptiveness.

Am I expecting too much of young people today? For the sake of this country, I hope not.

*   *   *

"Don't ask silly questions!" he shouted. "Why don't you go over to the hen house and cackle with the other old hens?" (The hen house was Joe's name for the clutch of elderly ladies who gathered after dinner to chat and gossip.)

Annie replied, "Well, if that's the way you feel, why do you manage to roost with them so often?" (It was generally known that Joe liked to pull up his chair and chat with the ladies.)

February 28, 1985

The new resident, also in a wheelchair, asked "How long have you been in this so-called home?"

I answered, "A little over five years."

Over five years," he repeated. "Why haven't you demanded that your family take you home?"

My first impulse was to tell him to mind his own business. Realizing he was expressing his pent-up hurts and emotions, I said, "I have no 'family,' as I believe you use the word, and no close relatives, and as I'm unable to care for myself, I live here and consider this my home."

"You've certainly let yourself be pushed around," he interrupted. "I can't take care of myself either, but if any of my free-loading relatives think they're going to relegate me to any institution for any length of time, they'd better rethink their priorities. My relatives aren't close either; they only think they are! Right now I've a mind to disinherit every last one of them. Even now, some of them will get quite a surprise when my last will is read."

Not wanting to get embroiled in any family situation, I suggested we go to the TV room and watch the news. En route, I thought, *Perhaps he'll soon come to terms with himself, his family, and his handicap.*

Observing the determined look on his face, I didn't feel too hopeful that the solution to his complaints would be permanent.

March 2, 1985

Joi de vivre—The French idiom that so happily expresses the quality of life we all want and seek.

Among his many worth-remembering comments, Norman Cousins said that the qualify of life was all-important and that each of us had the responsibility of controlling the quality of our own life.

I remember reading that or his words to that effect and thinking how I could better improve the quality of my life. I settled upon the following:

1. Try to eat and exercise sensibly (as much as I'm physically able).
2. Laugh a lot—mostly at myself when I can manage it.

3. Cry a bit for others' plights—not mine.

4. Try to love everyone—well, try to like most people; at least find something good in each. (There is always something good if you look for it.)

5. Try to keep busy. If physical activity is beyond me, then I learn something new to think about each day.

6. Try to be useful to someone.

7. Treasure friendships and happy memories.

8. Maintain my faith. If I do so, I don't believe my hopes will ever diminish.

I've tried to keep the above tenets, and while I can't say I've achieved *joi de vivre,* I can say I look forward to each new day with some degree of anticipation.

March 3, 1985

Speaking of anticipation, I'm looking forward to again hearing the Vienna Boys' Choir. COTG has arranged for those of us who are interested to attend the Powell Hall appearance of the choir Tuesday evening, March 5. I'm really quite excited about going.

I remember so well the first time I heard the choir. It was in Vienna many years ago. Hearing those clear young voices and watching their fresh young faces left me misty-eyed throughout the concert.

The second time I heard them I was en route home from Europe aboard the *Liberte.* The Boys' Choir was on board, too, going to the States to fulfill a program of personal appearances. The boys sang for the passengers at the captain's dinner. Everyone was captivated by them!

Tuesday evening I'll hear them in person for the third time, and I am grateful for the opportunity.

Leafing through the *Dial,* KETC/Channel 9's monthly magazine, I find the month of March is filled with interesting and beautiful things to see and hear on radio and TV. I've made a note of the following so that I'll be certain to tune in:

March 15—*Rigoletto* with Luciano Pavarotti.

March 17—*Man and Dolphins*—a documentary, filmed in the Bahamas, showing the *mutual exchange of information* between man and these fascinating creatures.

March 21—A skating spectacular—perhaps a preview in that category for the 1988 Olympics?

March 24—A gala of stars, including Beverly Sills and James Levine as host.

March 20—A two-hour tribute to Rodgers and Hammerstein, during which music from the following shows will be featured: *Oklahoma, The Sound of Music, The King and I, Carousel,* and *Flower Drum Song.* And to think I had the good fortune to see each one of those shows on Broadway—and each with the original cast.

How much I'd like to look over my old *Playbills.* I had kept all of them. Each was marked with the date, the name of the person or persons with whom I'd attended the performance, and usually my comments regarding the show.

Like so many things I haven't been able to locate since I broke up my home, I'll just dismiss them as lost and rely upon my memory to recall those pleasurable evenings.

March 27—*Tosca* from the Met with Hildegard Behrens and Placido Domingo.

And there are other interesting events I should add to my March agenda. I don't want to overlook the beautiful Bach music that KWMU is playing and will continue to play during this, the tercentenary of Johann Sebastian Bach's birth in 1685.

I respond emotionally to Bach's music, but I'm the first to confess I know nothing about the technicalities of counterpoint, of which he was the master, or so I'm told.

With so many interesting events coming up, I can see where March is going to be a month to be enjoyed.

March 4, 1985

I suppose everyone has his or her comeuppance at some time or other. I had mine today:

First, I was accused by an aide of saying something to her which I absolutely did *not* say.

Second, the COTG director, who heard the accusation and my denial, said I was condescending and that was probably the reason I was now unable to find a private duty aide who suited me.

No doubt she's right. I set high standards for myself and expect the best of others. When people don't measure up to their capabilities, I am disappointed. However, I wasn't aware that I was treating my disappointment as condescension. If that is so, then it's time I took me in hand!

Third, the therapist, shortly after the above confrontation, said she heard Mrs. Bennett had been in to see me. I answered, "Yes, she returned the journal entries which she had so graciously typed."

I continued, saying another friend of mine at UMSL had offered to type the balance of the entries.

The therapist replied that since I was giving scholarships to UMSL, she could understand the offer to help me.

Once when the therapist and I were discussing education in general, I told her how strongly I felt about kids receiving an education and that following my husband's death I had arranged to leave scholarship money in his name at the University of Missouri–Columbia and I was seriously considering doing the same for UMSL.

After this, I'll keep my intentions to myself. Better yet, I'll keep my mouth shut. I'm only sorry she put a dollar sign or value on my friends' offer to help.

As she was leaving my room, the therapist said she knew I was angry. I replied that she was wrong. I wasn't angry, but I was very hurt.

Last, to add to this unpleasant day, my COTG monthly bill has just been delivered to me.

I'm glad I'm still able to laugh—this time at the timing of the delivery. If the timing had been planned, it couldn't have been better.

March 5, 1985

Yesterday was a zero day—a real bummer. I couldn't find any elasticity in my bootstraps or any justification for the day's happenings.

I know now it is time I face reality, and the reality is, I've had a one-sided love affair with COTG. For over five years, I have mentally and emotionally as well as physically made it my "home." I had also let myself care too much.

I believe I know human nature well enough to understand the comments made by the aide and the therapist.

It was the director's remarks, made in front of others, that deflated my pride and/or vanity and diminished her in my eyes as the paragon administrator I thought her to be. Both hurt.

Much as I'd like to think otherwise, I have sense enough to know that my "loss of face" played no small part in upsetting my stomach to the point where I was afraid to attend the Boys' concert—an evening I had been anticipating.

It's not my deformed foot or surgical boots but my feet of clay that trip me. I must make more effort to remember that.

March 7, 1985

I needed a change of pace today and found it while leafing through the pages of the March issue of *Imprint,* a fashion forecast magazine published by Neiman-Marcus.

I'm intrigued with the article "Improbable Companions." Written with tongue in cheek, it lists the following names and items to stress the point of individualism: "Nancy Reagan, Mr. T., velvet, spandex and Madras Plaid and Boy George. It seems we'll be eclectic this spring if we'd be fashion-wise. It's avant guard and Hoi Polloi all in a melting pot. It's leather and lace or personal style in an age of generics."

Reading the magazine took me back to my retailing days, when I found it fun to watch the creators and the couturiers in titillating the fashion taste of the public. No matter how superficial it seems now, it does give me something to think about other than my own hurt feelings.

March 9, 1985

After carefully analyzing the nuances of their remarks, I know the nursing director and therapist both believe the accusations of the therapy aide. It may be that the COTG director (administrator) believes them, too.

I hope to talk with the director, and if that is so (I'll soon know), then what?

1. Do I make arrangements to move to another home? Because the truth is a matter of honor with me and this is the first time in my life my veracity has ever been questioned, *and I don't like it!*

or

2. Do I fall back on my faith, knowing eventually "truth will out."

I'll decide which after I talk with the director, who will be away for a couple of days.

March 11, 1985
The director is still away. However, the aide's accusations the other day caused me to do considerable soul searching, as well as an in-depth analysis of my environment, both physical and human.

More than my hurt feelings and pride, more than my concern as to whether or not I'm believed (the girl's own shortcomings will take care of that), is the realization that I need another environment.

Whether it's another home, an apartment of my own, or what, I only know I need a change! I'm hungry for stimulating conversation and companionship. My room is pleasant enough, but the hall on which I live falls short.

Little distinction has been made over the last few months in housing the handicapped—from the almost-total-care, somewhat-alert, from the wandering Alzheimers, et cetera, et cetera, et cetera. Up to this point, I've told myself, "Try not to criticize; you may be like that yourself someday."

If I am, *please, please* put me with my own ilk. *Please* don't burden someone other than that with me.

March 12, 1985
Death is not uncommon in a nursing home. Last weekend COTG lost a very gallant lady. Elizabeth knew she was terminal when she came here.

Her life had been one of adversity—there had been many operations, the loss of her youngest son through drowning, and an accident that left a handsome, very bright thirteen-year-old grandson mentally handicapped. The youth is now in his early twenties and attending an expensive "special school" in the East. I met the lad (clean-cut and quite handsome) on one of his trips home and could well understand Elizabeth's heartbreak.

Elizabeth confided in me once; otherwise I would never have known all she has experienced. She was always upbeat and I admired her greatly.

When her two sons told me, a few days ago, how much they appreciated my kindness to their mother, I could only say, "Thank you. Elizabeth always gave more than she received," and I meant it.

March 15, 1985

The Ides of March 1985.

So much has happened in the last few days, and as I seem to have thoughts about everything, I have some catching up to do.

1. There's the Russian succession. (Just when I learn to pronounce one name, the leadership changes.)
2. The evacuation of the American embassy personnel from Cypress to Beirut.
3. The 150th anniversary of Mark Twain's birth (Samuel Clemens, born 1835). I wouldn't have thought of that, but I heard it mentioned on TV and radio.
4. The visit of Highcroft Ridge School children to COTG yesterday. This is hardly in the same league with the Russian hierarchy or Beirut, but more pleasant to think about.

Regarding all the above, I'll jot down my unorganized thoughts as they occur to me. Now I may as well join the millions of other people around the world and speculate on what impact Gorbachev's leadership will have on the arms talks, the U.S.–USSR relationship, and overall world peace.

While speculating on that, I'll take time out to wonder what the new Egyptian ownership of Harrods will be like. Being old and conservative myself, I can only hope that fine old London store, known the world over, will not have too many of its traditions altered. (Whether you wanted an elephant, a perfect blue-white diamond, a drafty castle, or a whole smoked Scottish salmon, Harrods could and would get it for you.)

I remember the store best when Sir Richard Burbidge and Mr. Rodney Leathes were co-directors. That was before the Frazier regime.

I haven't been to London or in Harrods since I retired in 1974. I wonder if the huge chandelier, made of lead crystal goblets (and weighing a ton or two), is still hanging in shimmering beauty in the

customer dining room. I may never see it again, but I'll always re-
member it—as well as a letter from Rodney Leathes when I was trying
to track down a particular kind of caftan for an SBF customer. When
I was in doubt as to where to ferret out an obscure item for SBF's
"Round the World" shopping service, I'd contact Mr. Leathes at
Harrods.

His letter to which I'm referring told me where he believed I
could find "that Nigerian nightshirt." He was right and I was able to
purchase it for an SBF customer.

March 16, 1985

Regarding Beirut, I find it difficult to reconcile that war-ravaged,
devastated Beirut I see on TV with the beautiful Mediterranean city
I visited in 1967. It was known then as "The Paris of the Middle
East." I was first made personally conscious of the age-old conflict
between Arabs and Jews—but I'm getting ahead of my story. I'll
backtrack to Tel Aviv, where I had flown from Athens, Greece, a
week or so earlier.

I landed in Tel Aviv the first day of the 1967 Six-Day War. The
Israelis had shot down six Syrian planes that first day. As I recall,
Mr. and Mrs. J. A. Baer arrived the day after and when Mr. Baer
learned of the happenings of the previous day, he jestingly said to
Mrs. Baer and me, "If either of you hear any shooting, drop to the
ground. I'll be under you to soften the fall."

To proceed from Tel Aviv to Beirut as I planned to do within the
next few days, I found it necessary to fly via Nicosia, Cypress, as no
Israeli planes were permitted to land in Lebanon. In Nicosia I transferred to Mid-East Airlines, and proceeded on to Beirut, where I
landed at the beautiful new Beirut airport.

While in Beirut, I was taken as a guest to its noted casino, where
I saw a spectacular show, one worthy of the Folies Bergere.

I was fortunate to be in Beirut over a weekend and saw a more
spectacular sight when I took a Sunday tour to the ancient ruins of
Baalbek, the temple dedicated to the sun god, Baal, located in south-
west Syria.

*March 16, 1985,*P.M.

After hearing Mark Twain's name mentioned the other day, I
reread Dr. Lawrence Peters's sketch of him. This sketch contains

many of the humorist's pithy remarks. I remembered many of them; some I'd forgotten. All are worth requoting. Here are a few: "Man is the only animal that blushes—or needs to." "I have never let my schooling interfere with my education." "The man who doesn't read good books has no advantage over the man who can't read them." "I am different from George Washington, I have a higher standard of principle. He couldn't tell a lie. I can, but won't."

I know some libraries ban Twain's books because they think he's a racist. Perhaps a recent unearthed letter from him to Yale University will help dispel some of that feeling. In the letter he offers to pay for the schooling of a black boy, who later became a recognized lawyer.

The youngsters from Highcroft Ridge School visited us this week. Highcroft School is in nearby Chesterfield, Missouri. My little friend or pen pal is a delightful third-grader. A program for youngsters and oldsters getting together is jointly sponsored by the school and COTG.

The third-grade students accompanied by the school principal and a couple of their teachers periodically visit and entertain with group singing, dancing, and student solos. Following that, we chat and share punch and cookies. Later we correspond.

My little pen pal keeps me busy answering her letters and thanking her for the drawings and cut-out pictures she sends me. She's a joy, as were the two little boys who wrote to me a couple of years ago and the little girl who was my pen pal last year. I have some of this year's letters and artwork mounted on the back of one of my doors.

I know the youngsters bring us pleasure, and I believe the students gain a measure of practical knowledge from us.

March 17, 1985

I watched and admired her as she made her way among the tables at the Saint Patrick's Day party this afternoon. She extended a word of greeting here, a smile and a pat on the shoulder there. The residents all responded smilingly or with a pleasant comment. She looked tired. *No wonder,* I thought. The director's absence from COTG had been due to illness. I only asked her if she'd spare a few minutes for me when her busy schedule permitted. Perhaps this coming week? She graciously agreed. I continued watching her, all the while thinking, *Any good executive (like an admired and loved mother) wears many hats, but being the director of a nursing home,*

I have a feeling I should put this director back on her pedestal.

March 19, 1985

Unless you're restricted to two body positions (sitting up and lying down) and unless you've sat in a wheelchair (which is restrict-ive, too) for hours on end, I don't believe you'll fully realize how very tired your body can become.

Yesterday was a full day for me. Emily B——, who is always so considerate, took me to the dentist. We then had luncheon at the nearby Women's Exchange. Following that, she took me to buy a new pair of orthopedic shoes. We then went to the Lehyde Or-thopedic Company to have my brace transferred to the new shoe. Due to the backlog of work at Lehyde's, I'll not be able to pick up my new brace-shoe for a day or so.

By the time I returned to COTG, just in time to freshen up for supper, which I hardly touched, I was beginning to fold. It was 7:00 P.M. before anyone was free to help me lie down, and by then I was really bushed. Eight and a half hours in a wheelchair can be a mite tiring.

Today is Nell D——'s, Helen K——'s, and Zane S——'s birth-day. Each is a valued friend and I'll call each to extend my heartfelt wishes.

March 19, 1985, P.M.

A house doctor, a Dr. Cardiff, stopped by to see how Sarah was feeling. He said jovially, "Hello, Sarah. Do you know who I am?" Sarah replied, "Oh, good grief, don't you even know who you are?"

For the first time in almost five years, I'm beginning to see a glimmer of light at the end of the tunnel. I wore my new brace-shoe for the first time this morning. I was able to take a few steps in a shoe that even looks like a shoe and not a hunting boot. I'm deter-mined I'm going to make it this time! Not that I'll be able to walk normally, but I'll be able to take steps comfortably wearing a brace and using a cane as I did when I first came to COTG. This won't come overnight. But it will come!

I'll always be grateful to a young therapist by the name of Chris who worked with my foot so tirelessly. I give him full credit for starting me on the road back after my foot had reverted to the classic badly twisted stroke position. All the therapists since have worked diligently to keep my foot muscles and tendons straight and strengthened. Their efforts, and the tendon surgery I had, I know will pay off.

March 22, 1985

Two of our wandering ladies were walking toward me as I was looking out of the large glass patio window, wishing it were warmer so that I could sit outside for a bit. As the ladies passed me, one of them flipped her fingers, one by one, over her lower lip, at the same time blowing hard and using her tongue and lips to make a "pth-s-s-pthz-z-z" sound that startled me. I asked, "Was that meant for me?" "Oh, no," was the airy reply from one of the ladies, and waving her arm she continued, "It's a ptsh-s-s-pthz-z-z world, don't you think?" I was inclined to say, "Yes," but before I could say anything, the two of them ambled on.

I wondered if that very descriptive sound was still called a raspberry. Whatever it is called today, I was glad it wasn't meant for me exclusively.

March 23, 1985

My vagabond thoughts are footloose this morning. They're flitting from Pavarotti to the hoped-for meeting between President Reagan and Secretary General Gorbachev to Nuvo (that's fashion jargon for easy-to-wear clothes that say "wit" and carry a deft touch—it's primarily dressing to please the wearer) to the regular changing of the guard (nurse-aide-wise) here at COTG.

I realize "around-the-clock" care means three eight-hour shifts of nurses and aides each day seven days a week. All employees work a regular forty-hour, five-day week, which means each is entitled to two days off each week. To give all staff members a fair chance for "weekends off," days off are scheduled on different days each week.

I've often thought what a nightmare it must be for the person scheduling "days off." How do you please each aide and at the same time please each resident who has grown accustomed to the aide regularly assigned to that resident's hall? How? I don't know, but I wonder if an "understudy" program, such as used in the theater, might be feasible. I can see possibilities.

I lose my patience when for three shifts in a row I have an inexperienced aide who bumps and twists my sore-as-a-boil foot. It's about then I feel like spitting in someone's eye.

But to get back to Pavarotti. I couldn't manage his personal appearance at the Arena on the twenty-first, but I did manage to listen in on a rehearsal of the Kirkwood "Sweet Adeline" held at COTG on that evening. It was hardly a substitute, but nevertheless enjoyable.

As for the summit talk between Reagan and Gorbachev, I thought the recent remarks of Armand Hammer most encouraging. Hammer, who has had as much or more contact over the years with the Soviets than any other living American, feels the meeting is within the realm of possibility and that it might even take place in September when the UN convenes, if Gorbachev comes to the U.S. then.

Still March 23, 1985, 1:30 P.M.

If only one could inculcate, instill, or just plain pound into the heads of *some* of our young people that a job well done carries with it more than financial pay. There's pride of accomplishment, self-satisfaction, and even pleasure. Added benefits accrue when one does more than expected. Going that extra mile, whether it's in your job or helping another, brings about self-fulfillment that is beyond dollar remuneration.

Earlier today the therapy aide came to my room to tell me she had confused my name with that of another resident and that she realized how unfair she had been in accusing me. I accepted her apology, but told her I'd appreciate it if she'd explain her error to Mrs. Bono. She said she would.

March 24, 1985

It has been a ten plus day—a beautiful Sunday.

After a relaxing whirlpool bath, I'm now in bed, reflecting upon the day's happenings while watching and listening to Beverly Sills, James Levine, and their gala of stars. It has been a diversified program, with everything from Bach and Debussy, a cello solo, and Levine playing the piano to Domingo and Merill to Gershwin's "I've Got Rhythm," just to name a few of the features.

The day started off just so-so, but gained momentum when I had a good brace-shoe-quad-cane walk.

In the afternoon, one of my favorite people, Ken W——, spent a couple of hours with me. It's always such a pleasure when he stops by. Ken is intelligent, extremely well read, and very stimulating. He and Eve raised and college-educated three fine kids, and I love to hear about them.

Today I heard about Larry, their younger son, a very bright young attorney. He graduated from law school about three or four years ago; he took and passed both the Missouri and the Arizona bar. He and his young wife, Claudia, then spent a year in Japan. Upon his return to the U.S., he became an Arizona county attorney. (I don't recall the name of the county, but it's the one in which the Grand Canyon is located.) Today, after resigning from his county position and spending several days with his parents in St. Louis, he and Claudia boarded a plane for Fort Lee in Virginia, where he will take basic military training and join the adjutant general's staff. Then he goes to Europe, where he'll practice law as a military lawyer.

March 25, 1985

The COTG director and I have just concluded a pleasant and, I believe, mutually satisfactory talk.

Because I felt I owed her the courtesy of telling her I planned to leave COTG, I spelled out my reasons why and how I had arrived at the decision. She, in turn, convinced me she had been placed in a very difficult position, et cetera (which I did and do understand). She asked if I would consider moving into the new wing of this facility, which is currently under construction. I said I would consider such a move.

In short, as far as I'm concerned, the entire "aide" matter is a closed issue, at least at the present.

March 27, 1985

When Ken W—— visited me the other day, he returned a little pocket notebook in which I had annotated the itinerary and highlights of a foreign trip I made in 1969. Ken had been a member of a buying committee of which I, as a merchandise manager, was the "mama-san."

Briefly, Associated Dry Goods Corporation, owner of many of the better known department stores in the U.S. (including such stores as Lord and Taylor of New York, Hornes of Pittsburgh, SBF of St. Louis, Robinson's of Los Angeles, et cetera) sent many of their buyers abroad to buy foreign merchandise. Because I had made many trips for SBF to Europe, the Middle East, and the Far East, I was asked by ADG on several occasions to act as counselor for committees of buyers from member stores to buy for certain departments that I had merchandised or was merchandising at the time.

On this particular 1969 trip, I worked with a group of buyers in Europe—then I flew to the Orient to work with a different group of ADG buyers, who were to meet me in Tokyo.

Leafing through the notebook this morning brought back many memories of tiring but happy workdays and quite a few humorous incidents.

On this 1969 jaunt, I worked with two three-buyer committees where each buyer represented a department that I had at some time or other merchandised.

The European Committee was comprised of Ken W—— from SBF, Jane L——, a young woman from Stewarts of Baltimore, and Dick B—— of Denver Dry Goods of Colorado. They were hardworking, knowledgeable, and thoroughly delightful people. I enjoyed every minute I was with them.

The four of us met on February 22, 1969, at Kennedy Airport in New York and took off that evening for Frankfort, Germany, where we planned to attend the Frankfort Trade Fair.

After working the Frankfort fair and spending a few hours at the Offenbach fair, just across the river Maine from Frankfort, we flew to Nuremburg for a couple of days, then on to London where we spent a week shopping the market and visiting stores like Harrods, Fortnum and Mason, Liberty House, et cetera.

On the Sunday before leaving London for Italy, we spent most of the day sightseeing. I had made several trips to London and knew a bit about "Old London Towne," but Ken had lived several years in London and knew his way around far better than I.

The others on the committee and I took advantage of his knowledge and visited Petticoat Lane, London Bridge and Tower, the House of Lords, the House of Commons, Westminster Abbey (complete with organ music), the Parliament Building, Buckingham Palace, Parade Grounds, Pall Mall, and St. James Castle.

Hungry, weary, and history-satisfied (for the moment), we ended up at the Grosvenor House for something to eat. I don't know if we ever decided if it was for an extremely late, late luncheon or for a very early supper.

The next day we flew to Rome and took the train to Florence, where we were to spend several days. After the second day, I left the committee in Florence and took the *Rapido* to Rome, where I stayed overnight at the Excelsior. I left the next day on Lufthansa as scheduled. The plane made its first scheduled stop in Cairo, where I watched Egyptian soldiers atop sandbags around the airport taking pot shots at a plane overhead. I assumed it was an Israeli plane, but I had no way of really knowing.

The second scheduled stop was made in Kuwait; however, upon takeoff there, the #2 engine caught fire. The pilot aborted the takeoff—how, I don't know. I was told later by the crew that it was nearly a serious accident and that only a very good pilot could have avoided it.

The continuing flight to Bangkok, an intermediate stop on my way to Tokyo, was canceled. Three and a half hours later, with the help of the Lufthansa crew, I was able to get on an Air India plane for Bangkok, via Bombay and New Delhi. I arrived in Bangkok nine and a half hours late.

Having missed connections, reservations, and everything else I could think of, I stayed overnight at the Siam International, which was close to the airport. In Bangkok, I usually stopped at the Oriental, Mandarin, or Dusit Thani. That night I would have found a park bench comfortable.

The next morning I was able to get out on Air France to Tokyo, *but* via Saigon, where I could hear artillery fire from the airport. (The Vietnam War was still in full swing.)

I finally arrived in Tokyo late that night and checked into the Palace Hotel. The committee members had waited up for me, and I started out to work the next morning with my new committee. What a roundabout way to reach Tokyo!

March 28, 1985

Is it old age, frustration, the eighty-nine-degree heat this March day, just plain cussedness, or a soupçon of each?

Whatever it is, I know I became increasingly irritable as this day wore on. The little annoyances that I wouldn't have dignified with a second thought before my stroke are now making me cross and grumpy. Think I'll go to bed and forget the last few hours. Tomorrow will be a better day!

Four hours later, March 29, 1985, in bed, asleep or was

Tomorrow will be a better day? Who sez?

The metal side rail on my hospital bed just dropped down with a bang and clatter that scared the "bejayzus" out of me. Now, if I can go back to sleep and stop shaking, I'll try to see the humor in this early morning drama later.

March 30, 1985

What a difference a day makes—or shouldn't make! Yesterday was pretty much of a bust, but I'd managed to laugh everything off up to and including breakfast this morning. Even the rain that started today off on two left feet and my gloomy tablemates at breakfast didn't bother me. Then what did? In thinking over the events of the last twenty-four hours, I believe the thing that upsets me most and makes me the most impatient is the lack of just plain common sense that afflicts so many people.

I don't expect weighed judgments from too many, and I certainly don't expect academic knowledge (we all know too many "educated fools" for that), but a little common sense, even of the horse variety, is it too much to expect? And what brought forth this outburst?

I asked the aide who was making my bed this morning to be certain to leave my call light cord where I could reach it from my wheelchair. She assured me that she would. When I returned from breakfast, I found the call light cord behind the bed. I spent thirty minutes of time and energy trying to fish it out with my quad cane. I couldn't make it. Finally, hearing the voice of one of the housekeepers in the hallway, I opened the door and asked if she'd give me a hand. A small annoyance, perhaps, and one I should probably

overlook, but I think too many people
walk but don't bother to look,
look but don't bother to see,
hear but don't bother to listen,
listen but don't even try to comprehend, and unfortunately
talk and act without thinking.

P.S. How pedantic the above sounds. It even irks me—and how condescending it must sound to others.

March 31, 1985

Palm Sunday—cloudy and chilly damp. A good day to stay indoors. A good day for reflection, contemplation, and anticipation.

Reflecting upon many of the past experiences that have contributed to my development and brought me to this place in time, I find that with every experience there has always been a lesson—something for me to learn and ponder over, something to add to my growth and I hope to my stature.

Even unhappy experiences have taught me to discard useless mental activity such as sorrow, disappointment, even discouragement. Because I cannot hold two opposite thoughts in my mind *at the same time*, I don't find it too difficult to crowd out of my mind any negative, destructive, or pessimistic thoughts by persistently holding in my mind the opposite—the positive, constructive, and optimistic thoughts.

Contemplating what experience has taught me, I find that now:

1. I don't mourn over lost opportunities. Instead I set up new goals.
2. I don't grieve over past mistakes. Instead I try very hard never to repeat the same mistake.

Anticipating isn't too difficult—this being Holy Week and with Easter coming up representing renewal, resurgence, and reawakening! It's a time to discard hurtful habits and hurt feelings. It's a time to take on new attitudes.

The miracle of Easter isn't something that happened that day of resurrection two thousand years ago. Easter continues for me whenever I'm receptive to renewal with better ideas and attitudes.

* * *

At this moment, I'd love to be in Italy! I've been watching the NBC telecast from Rome. It brought back a rush of memories of that friendly country. Italians are the only people I know who can laugh, cry, and sing all at the same time.

Italy has been so much in my thoughts lately. It was only last week that Gerry B—— and her son Rick left St. Louis for a four-week sojourn in Italy.

Were I a bit farther along in my restorative therapy, I'd take off right now for Rome—wheelchair and all. First, I'd call Stuart Hartzell, once manager of Alitalia in St. Louis. He's now or was head of his own travel agency, Montclair. Anyway, I'd start making reservations somewhere; I'd call an agency, hire a nurse aide, and before long I'd be on my way.

I'll just dream for now, but God willing, sometime within the next few years, I'm going to manage one or more of these missed and longed-for trips.

Today I'll just think about Rome, the Spanish Steps, the Vatican, the Bascilica, Bulgaris, and the fashionable Via Condotti, Trevi Fountain, the Coliseum, the colorful carabinieri and their rooster-plumed hats, the Forum, Via Veneto, et cetera, et cetera. From Rome I'd take the Rapido to Florence, that fabulous city. What memories I have of the Ponte Veccio, the Arno, Mario V——, his charming family, and the many pleasant hours I spent with them. The only time I heard Furtwangler in person and the Berlin Philharmonic was in Florence. It was my birthday and I was the guest of Renato Mosca, then head of the AMC Italian office. Furtwangler had the most expressive hands I've ever seen on any human being. If I remember correctly, he was killed in an auto accident in the Black Forest of Germany shortly after that appearance in Florence. I've always been glad that I had the opportunity to see and hear him.

Then to Milan (La Scala), the Milan Cathedral, et cetera. On to Lake Como and Villa d'Este, over to Venice (St. Mark's Square, the Rialto and Grand Canal, and the wind-swept Adriatic) and of course nearby Murano. I wouldn't forget Naples and the hydro-planes to the Isle of Capri, and I'd certainly not overlook Sardinia and Sicily. I can conjure up enough Italian sights and memories to last me a lifetime. Right now, it's 8:30 A.M. and time to go to the COTG dining room for breakfast. From Rome, Italy, to Ballwin, Missouri—a sizable jump mile-wise but not memory-wise.

April 3, 1985

Helen and Joel K—— spent yesterday afternoon with me—and Emily B—— and Zen S—— stopped by last evening. I can't help thinking what wonderful friends I have. Hardly a day goes by that someone doesn't phone. And often during the week or on a weekend, a friend or two will take the trouble to stop by and spend an hour or so with me.

Just a few days ago, Barbara and Ed F—— stopped by to tell me of their planned trip to Europe in May. They'll take a boat through the canals of Holland, then fly on to Paris. From France they intend to spend some time in Switzerland. Helen and Joel are knee-deep in travel plans, too.

What fun I'm going to have traveling vicariously this year.

April 4, 1985

Following my orthopedist's instructions, I have worn a custom-made plastic foot/leg cast every night while sleeping for the last four months. The cast is to train and strengthen my foot muscles and tendons.

While waiting for adjustments to be made on my new brace-shoe, I have worn, for a couple of mornings, the plastic cast to breakfast. That started rumors. The feedback tells me I have everything from a twisted ankle to smashed toes and a broken foot to arterial surgery. I wouldn't be at all surprised to hear I have hoof and mouth disease.

The gossip is amusing in a way and not so funny in another. Oldsters, I know, need to express ourselves in some manner. It's regrettable if that expression takes the form of gossip. In this instance, the gossip is amusing and harmless. There are times, however, when gossip can be hurtful.

April 7, 1985

I was asked today, "What is your religion? What do you believe?"

I doubt if I can succinctly express or explain what I so firmly believe. However, I'll try. One hears, reads, or says "superpowers," and immediately most people first think, *The United States and Russia.*

I believe there is only one superpower and that is that power that created and continues to create the life force that is in every living organism. To my knowledge, with all his scientific know-how, man has never been anything but a manipulator where life force is concerned. For example, man can take a tulip bulb and plant, fertilize, and nurture it. When it flowers, he'll probably pat himself on the back for growing a beautiful tulip, but man has never been able to duplicate the life force within that bulb. Neither has he duplicated the life force within an acorn that eventually produces a giant oak tree.

Nor has he been able to duplicate the life force within the sperm and the egg. Man merely manipulates the two to produce a test-tube baby.

That precious life force is within each of us. How we nurture and guide that life force determines the direction of our lives.

The use of that superpower-given force (I prefer to say God-given life force) by Christ and the faith of his followers in Christ's words, actions, and deeds became the foundation of Christianity.

Christianity took off in many directions, but few (if any) religious beliefs *disavow* a power (whatever the name) greater than finite man.

That belief in a superpower is the basis of my faith.

April 8, 1985

I am appalled at the statistics I just read. These figures were released by the Association of American Geographers and the National Council for Geographic Education. The article declared the United States is fast becoming "a nation of Geographic Illiterates."

The report also cited a 1983 test in geography developed by prominent educators and administered by the *Dallas Times Herald* to American twelve-year-olds.

More than 20 percent of the students couldn't locate the United States on a world map. Another 20 percent identified Brazil as the United States. The report went on to say that in a college-level survey on global understanding by the Educational Testing Service, the media score was an appalling 42.9 out of a possible 100!

To me it seems impossible to properly evaluate a world event without an understanding of geographic relationships. How can one grasp the importance of the Sinai Peninsula in Egyptian-Israeli relations when one believes the Sinai to be in Vietnam? (This and many other incredible answers have turned up in recent government surveys.)

I think geographic illiteracy is but a reflection of today's home and school standards. Listen to the grammar and the English used by many Americans and you'll think as I do, that we've raised not one, but at least two generations of illiterates, not only in geography, history, and grammar, but in just about everything else you can think of that makes for a well-rounded, educated person. Amen! Now I'll shut up and stop preaching.

April 12, 1985

As time goes by (and certainly a lot of it has gone by me), I realize, more and more, how fortunate I've been all of my life. Even my stroke treated me more gently than a severe stroke treats many people. My mind was not affected, or so my friends tell me. Neither was my speech impaired, as I seem to chatter and carry on a conversation as before.

Oh, yes, I'd prefer it if my lopsided smile didn't try to slide off the left side of my face. And it certainly would be more convenient if my left hand and arm could be used for something other than to anchor a table napkin on my lap.

But my left foot, even though still very tender and often hurtful, each day seems to be slipping more easily into my brace-shoe, and my walking (I should say mechanical-like stepping) seems to be more comfortable with each step.

All of my past, fortunate and unfortunate, has taught me to live each day moment by moment, hour by hour, until each day becomes a fulfilled learning experience.

April 14, 1985

For the past two or three weeks, I've had the feeling that my paralyzed foot wasn't responding to the physical therapy I am undergoing. Yesterday, my foot appeared to me to be reverting back to the twisted classic stroke position it had reverted to once before.

Fearful of that, I carefully watched every movement, voluntary and involuntary, that my foot made or that was made to it. After careful observation, I concluded that the heavy leather strap that positions my foot on the pedal of the bicycle I ride every day for fifteen or twenty minutes was twisting my foot and I believe negating some of the beneficial effects of my labored brace-shoe walking.

Testing my theory, I didn't ride the bicycle today. I found I was then able to keep my brace-shoe on after walking much longer today than yesterday. Too, my foot, following walking, felt much better than it did yesterday.

April 15, 1985

Watching "60 Minutes" last evening and hearing again about communist Albania and the recent death of Hoxha, the dictator these many years of that beautifully scenic but isolated, backward country, recalled to my mind the many interesting conversations I had with Phyllis L——.

Phyllis was a resident here when I first arrived at COTG in December 1979. We were tablemates in the dining room for many months prior to her death from congestive heart failure.

While neither one of us had ever been to Albania, we had some interesting discussions and exchange of ideas. She was of Albanian descent and kept in close contact with the small Albanian community in St. Louis. She knew a great deal about that violent, war-torn little Balkan country. I only knew what I read in newspapers or history books. Albania was off-limits to U.S. citizens when I was doing most of my traveling.

Phyllis was intelligent and articulate, and I thoroughly enjoyed the time we spent together.

April 16, 1985

Someone once said, "When you are at the end of your rope, there are three things you can do: 1. You can let go. 2. You can tie a knot in the end of the rope and hang on. 3. You can splice the rope and begin again."

I've become quite adept at tying knots and even more adept at splicing, all because I learned a long time ago not to let go.

I learned, too, there's always a way to solve every problem. The way or the solution may take one of many forms:

1. Rethink the problem—it's usually less momentous than you thought. Sometimes it isn't there at all.
2. Define your options. There are often two or three alternatives, usually more attractive than the solutions you were so obstinately seeking.
3. Look beyond the problem. You'll find a larger view, which more times than not will alter your attitude and give you the courage to start over.

April 18, 1985

I watched the telecast from the Met last evening of *Simon Boccanegra* and went to sleep thinking of Venice, the Doge Palace, the Danielli, and Milnes's vibrant baritone and wondering why the story lines of most operas (grand and soap alike) are so complicated.

Later I realized that any one of the ordinary events of any day could be turned into an interesting story or developed into a complicated plot.

I wonder what a good storyteller would do with the following:

About an hour ago, I fumbled a bottle of my favorite perfume, spilling about a fourth of it. The perfume had been given to me by a long-time friend of Morgan's and mine.

A short time after my stroke, he asked me, wheelchair and all, to marry him, saying I would need someone to care for me now that Morgan was gone.

I knew then, and I suspect he did, too, that I would never remarry. I've often thought how grateful he must be whenever he reflects upon my refusal. I feel now as I did then that it wouldn't be fair to marry any man, as I'd probably always mentally compare him to Morgan. Too, I would never consciously inflict my crippled self and wheelchair on any man or, for that matter, any woman, friend, or relative.

The donor of the perfume understands, I'm certain, as we've remained good friends over the years.

April 19, 1985

She very carefully removed the beribboned, beflowered straw hat from the artfully decorated "Springtime" wall arrangement. She, one of our wandering ladies, looked into an imaginary mirror, patted her hair, pretended to powder her nose, moistened her lips, then placed the "springtime" bonnet on her head.

Two or three times she started to walk on when she saw me. She then hesitated, smiled, and blithely waved her hand. Returning her friendly greeting, I thought she looked quite pretty in her gayly decorated straw hat. Looking quite pleased with herself, she wandered on.

April 21, 1985, 9:30 A.M.

A beautiful day, I thought, as the sun streamed through my window. A *ten day,* I continued. Within thirty minutes, my ten day had plummeted to a zero day. Two hours later, I am now trying to put into practice my theories of rope splicing and problem solving.

If my theories work (and I know they will if I but try), I'll not enumerate the happenings that precipitated today's miserable start. Instead, I'll begin my splicing and solving by stating, "No one was or is to blame." The situation this morning arose from a series of conditions, past and present, both mine and the nursing home's. With that in mind, I'll begin my climb toward a ten day. Tonight when I go to bed, I'll be able to say, "I've made it a good day." So—until tonight.

April 21, 1985 (still) 9:00 P.M.

I didn't quite make it! My foot hurts too much, my stiff knee was too bothersome, and there were too many willing aides doing their best to help me all day long.

The regular hall aide on the day shift is on vacation, and the regular evening shift aide went home ill. All in all, eight different aides on the two shifts divided up the work, on and off, in getting me from bed, removing my leg/foot cast and arm splint, helping me dress, and putting on my brace-shoe.

In the evening the process was reversed in helping me to undress, giving me a whirlpool bath, putting on my night cast and splint, and helping me to bed. Right now, I don't think my foot could take another pull, twist, or bump. Instead of the ten day I was going to make it, it's turning out to be a two day for me physically and a seven day for me emotionally. The sincere efforts of the aides in trying to make me comfortable almost made it possible for me to succeed in reaching my goals. At the same time, those efforts kept it from becoming a ten day.

Doesn't make sense, does it?

April 22, 1985, 9:30 P.M.

Today started off no better than yesterday, but it's ending up being a ten day, all because Jean David asked her husband, Russ, to play a song I had long wanted to hear again. But let me explain:

Tonight was COTG's Coronation Ball, at which our selection of a nursing home queen was crowned. A Queen's Supper followed. Entertainment for the evening was provided by Russ David, John Becker, and Marty Bronson.

Jean David, who has been quite ill, is now a resident here at COTG. She was seated not too far from the piano. I was nearby. When Russ dedicated a couple of numbers, including "Always," to Jeannie, I'm afraid I choked up. About that time, Rusty, the Davids' oldest son, walked up, kissed his mother, and greeted me. Trying hard to swallow the lump in my throat, I asked if sometime he or his dad would play the composition of another well-known Russ. I asked for Russ Morgan's "Does Your Heart Beat for Me?," one of Morgan's and my favorites.

I wasn't aware that Jeannie had even heard my request, as she seemingly had been absorbed in her own thoughts and not paying much attention to anyone. However, she leaned over toward Russ and asked him to play the song I'd mentioned.

I was delighted for two reasons. First, Jeannie then appeared more alert, animated, and smiling than I had seen her in quite some time. As for me, the song brought back a flood of happy memories and the evening ended on a sentimental, nostalgic note.

April 23, 1985

I just heard from Cubby. He and Pat are celebrating their twentieth wedding anniversary in Europe. It doesn't seem possible that it has been twenty years since they married.

The two of them are now in London following a stay on the Continent. They first went to Munich, "saw Julius Baer [Carl's brother], who is unbelievable at 83." Then on to Baden Baden, past Pforzheim ("our old hang-out") over to Venice, and returning to Paris by "fabulous Orient Express."

While in Paris, they had luncheon with Renee Robrieux, and while in London, they will have luncheon with John and Betty Miller.

What wonderful memories Cub's words evoke—memories of happy working days, of European friends, and of the many times Cub's, Pat's, and my paths crossed while traveling abroad.

I recall Pat and Cub's honeymoon trip to Europe. They were just leaving Capri where Cub had taken ill. I was in Florence at the time when Cub called me, asking if I'd follow through on an idea he had about a little charm made by the artist David Rawnsley.

I went to Naples and took the hydroplane to Capri, where I met David and Phyllis Rawnsley. From that meeting the Capriti promotion was developed for SBF.

SBF ran an ad about the Capriti in the New Yorker. Requests for the little charm were received from every state in the union. Even some of the boys in Vietnam wrote asking for the charm.

I still have some of the promotional material and the story developed for the promotion. And I still have one of the many letters we received expressing the sentiment the little charm evoked. The story about the Capriti follows:

Capriti

Capriti are strange legendary creatures which inhabit the island of Capri. Variously described, they are part frog, part mouse, and part bird: A cross between a leprechaun and a gremlin. They are seldom seen except in the half light upon the mountainside and on the great cliffs of Monte Solaro. Local superstition credits them with magic powers, and few people dare leave the island without one or more small replicas which are regarded as talismans of great good fortune.

The trouble pots are small earthenware vessels in which the Capriti were supposed to live. It is said that troubles, once firmly sealed in the pots, can never again emerge, and the Capriti from then on will accompany their owners to guard them from harm and to advise them upon the personal problems of their lives.

According to the legend, a Sage once lived on the Isle of Capri. He was known far and wide for the infallible advice he gave to those who brought their troubles to him. His method was simple and effective: for a small sum, he gave, to those who sought his advice, a little earthenware pot. From this they withdrew the spirit of good fortune and peace of mind, which he called "capriti," and in its place they put their troubles, which they then dropped into the blue depths of the ocean, where they were lost forever. Relieved of their cares, they would leave, accompanied by their own special talisman, the Capriti, which would from then on protect them from further evil.

The miracle still works as it did of old. The magic of the Capriti is still as strong, providing they are cared for correctly. They live upon kind thoughts and deeds, and the more they receive of this nourishment the stronger does their magic become. Take one for your friend and one for your enemy and one for yourself. New friends will be made, old quarrels healed. When in difficulty or doubt, you have a friend at hand. Listen to his infallible advice, and, in your inner heart, you will hear his small, quiet voice showing you a way of life that will bless you, and those around you, as long as you live.

One of the Many Letters Received Regarding SBF's Capriti Promotion

Advertising Manager STIX BAER FULLER St. Louis, Missouri

Sir: It has taken me 38 years (20 of them as a professional writer) to give in (almost) to the people who've been telling me all this time what a bitchy, back-biting world we live and work in.

Due mainly to circumstances involving my family over the past two years, I had, finally, begun to wonder if maybe the pessimists weren't right after all. Syrupy as it may sound, I found my faith in people completely restored by your Capriti ad in the New Yorker. I was writing a check before I'd finished reading the copy.

But the thing I thought you might like to know is this: when the time came for me to put my troubles in the pot, I cut memo pad paper into fortune cookie–size strips . . . and couldn't think of a darned thing important enough to write down.

I did, hopefully, jot down some of the family problems . . . convinced that Capriti could work for people close to me as well as for me alone.

But I'd like the person responsible for the Capriti to know that it is truly heart-warming, in this age of space races and rat races, to know that someone took time to see, buy and write about something that is "part frog, part mouse, part bird, part myth" . . . and ALL heart.

Who knows? If it weren't for the atmosphere of kindness and affection in which Capriti must be nurtured . . . I might not be writing this letter at all!

Anyway . . . sincere thanks for the way the arrival of the captivating creatures brightened the day for everyone here at the agency. It's about time that troubles got potted instead of people!

There's only one drawback. I look for a terrible drop in the martini market.

> Regards,
> Pendleton Copywriter
> Botsford, Constantine McCarty

April 23 continued

Then there was the time Pat, Cub, and I met in Lisbon, where we had dinner at Avis, following which we went fadoing. At different times, there were dinners together in Athens, in Tel Aviv, in Paris.

There were many humorous incidents, too. One in particular I still chuckle over. Several retailers were en route to Europe on the *Queen Mary.* Cub and I were from SBF. There was a general merchandise manager and a buyer or two from Higbees, Cleveland, a buyer from Carson, Pirie Scott, Chicago, and a buyer or two from Neiman-Marcus, Dallas.

We arranged to have our meals together in the Veranda Room. It was a very pleasant, enjoyable crossing. The evening before we were to dock at Le Havre, Cub suggested we all meet the next morning in the lounge to be ready early for the French customs officials when they came aboard.

Next morning I was little bright eyes, up, packed, my luggage taken to the lounge, and was just ready to step out of my stateroom when my phone rang. It was Cub asking if I'd mind stopping by his stateroom on my way to the lounge.

The minute he opened his door, I knew why he wanted me to stop by. There, on the foot of his bed, was a piece of luggage piled high with clothing. Obviously, the case couldn't be closed. Cub asked if I'd mind sitting on top of the luggage while he tried to snap it shut. He hoisted me to the almost perpendicular top and finally succeeded in closing the case. I hopped down.

It was then we noticed a pile of soiled linen he had failed to have laundered and had forgotten to pack. Prior to our departure from New York, each of us had been given a bon voyage bottle of champagne, packed in a metal cannister from Saks, which had inscribed on it

NOBODY BUT NOBODY

It was a Saks slogan at the time. I had given my metal cannister to my steward, who had admired it. Cub still had his, so we packed as much of the linen in it as we could. The residual we packed in a discarded torn cardboard suit box, which Cub secured by strapping with one of his belts.

He, carrying the tin can, and I, carrying the belted bedraggled suit box, marched on to the lounge, greeted our friends, chatted with the French customs, disembarked, took the boat train to Paris, and registered at the Ritz Hotel. That was many years ago, and I know it didn't bother either one of us at the time that we looked like a couple of refugees who had just come over in steerage. We were only grateful everything held together and we didn't leave a trail of socks, shorts, and shirts.

April 24, 1985

I have just returned from an enjoyable luncheon at Garden Villas. Henry and Barbara Grossberg own several St. Louis nursing homes and retirement facilities—Garden Villas and Clayton on the Green being two of them.

This is the third year residents of Garden Villas have invited residents from their sister facilities to join them for luncheon. As usual, the food was delicious.

Le Menu
Asti spumanti
Ritz Crab or Tuna Bake
on
Toasted English Muffin
Julienne Carrots
Asparagus Spears
Chocolate Eclair
Coffee—Tea
Blums After-Dinner Mints

Following the luncheon, Russ David entertained at the keyboard. He spent almost two hours playing nostalgic songs long remembered by the residents, who responded with enthusiastic applause.

What impressed me most about the outing was that again COTG and its caring staff "bothered" to take more wheelchair residents than did the other facilities. I was first impressed by this fact when five local nursing homes took some of their residents to a "Pops" concert at Queeny Park. On this occasion, COTG had taken five residents with cumbersome wheelchairs. There was only one wheelchair among the other four facilities. All the other residents were ambulatory and far less "bother" than those in wheelchairs.

April 25, 1985

Many years ago on one of my buying trips to Europe, a small tradition was born in Paris. It was May Day. Ken Wilde and a young fellow buyer presented me with a bouquet of lilies of the valley. Since my retirement, the Wildes have given me a pot of growing lilies of the valley on May Day or as close to it as the fragrant flowering of the plant permits.

Today Ken again brought me their token of friendship. As always, I count their thoughtfulness among my many blessings.

April 28, 1985

The word "transmission" buried in the middle of the printed column caught my eye. I unfolded the newspaper to see these headlines:

LOTUS ETNA
WILL OFFER
WHIZ-BANG
TECHNOLOGY

Price will be $150,000.00
For super car due in 1988

I read on: "For the real future in innovative automation technology one might look to tiny Lotus cars, the British sports-car specialist and its sensational Etna show-car designed by Italy's Giugiaro."

The article goes on to say that if the Etna is any indication, future drivers should be able to navigate by satellite, park by sonar, and verbally command their radios to tune themselves to a favorite station.

The present Lotus car, officials say, is the forerunner of a new supercar that will be put into production by 1988 and will cost $150,000.00 Ultra high performance will be delivered by Etna's new 340 horsepower, four-liter V8, coupled to a continuously variable automatic transmission (which is like having an infinite number of gear ratios to maximize performance) and optional four-wheel drive, all controlled by computer.

Why, I thought, *would a handicapped female oldster residing in a nursing home be interested in any article such as this?*

Easy, I answered myself. *Because your father, Fred H. Ream, invented the ballbearing universal joint.*

That was back in 1900 something or other. I only know because I have a brochure from 1919 explaining the product. I have been told by people who should know that his ideas were the forerunner of the front-wheel drive.

A few years ago, I sent the original drawings and patent grants to my father's grand-nephew James D. Ream, Jr., who is an engineer with NASA and lives with his family on Merritt Island, Florida.

I thought as I read the article how interested Dad would be in it and what fun he'd have with the new technology. Unfortunately, he's missing all the new technological developments, because he died at almost ninety years of age in 1973, still as mentally alert as anyone I've ever known.

April 30, 1985

She said she could find no justification for her to go on living. If only she could end it all and relieve her family of the wearisome chore of coming to see her. Their attempts at cheering her only made her realize how empty her life was now and how useless it was to go on day after day dreading the dawn of each tomorrow—increasingly missing all that previously had been important to her. Oh, if she could just put a stop to these endless days.

I wanted to comfort her, but found her mind closed to everything but a return to the life she had once known.

From experience, I knew that was impossible. I knew, too, that only with an altered attitude could she find some degree of contentment with her illness and restricted life. I wanted to tell her that by taking certain steps she could achieve a much happier tomorrow:

1. Mentally *accept* her handicap.
2. Recognize it will *change* her life-style.
3. Make up her mind to *learn* and *grow* or at least *adjust* to each new alteration or change.
4. *Believe* there are many people who *care* and want to help her.
5. Be receptive.
6. Try all of the above and know that with every effort she'll strengthen her determination to keep on trying.

Surprisingly, the first thing she'll discover is that she'll stop longing for the past. Instead, she'll let her happy memories influence the way she looks at people and situations today. Soon she'll minimize the annoyances, hurts, frustrations, and dissatisfactions that dominate her life now. Before long those dissatisfactions will fade into the background. More important, her faith will be strengthened, and she'll realize God never placed on her shoulders more than she could handle. I know.

May 1, 1985

The last ten days have been disappointing. My foot continues to be sensitive and hurting. Too, my leg has started to buckle when I try to walk, even when wearing the steel brace I had altered at the suggestion of the therapist and physiatrist. I have the feeling I'm retrogressing again instead of progressing. While I'm no doctor, phys-iatrist, or therapist, I'm convinced something I'm wearing, using, or doing is working at cross purposes with my muscle/tendon training and therapy goals.

I'm not discouraged, but I am disappointed and no little annoyed that after six and a half years of hospital, doctor, surgeon, and therapy bills, I'm faced with starting over again.

Giving up has never been one of my propensities, so as usual, I'll say, "I'll make it," and I will.

I can hardly pronounce the word "physiatrist"—let alone spell it. Wonder if I did spell it correctly?

May 2, 1985

I sound like a broken record even to myself, but I know no better way to *keep me keeping on* than to remind myself that my deter-mination has paid off before and that it will again if I just *keep on keeping on.*

May 3, 1985

My third "beginning again" and a modicum of success. I walked about fifty feet this morning without my knee giving out. It's a start! I didn't quite make my goal of fifty feet today—but there's always tomorrow and tomorrow.

May 5, 1985

Today is Barbara and Ed Fick's fiftieth wedding anniversary. How I wish Morgan and I could have made it to fifty. We didn't, but our fortieth was heartwarming.

On November 26, 1977, I felt forty years was quite a milestone and I wanted to give Morgan something more than just a material gift. So in addition to some stereo components I knew he wanted, I wrote him a letter mentioning some of the highlights of forty years of happy marriage and telling him what those forty years had meant to me.

He told me that when he read my letter he realized it was the most precious gift he'd ever received.

Three months later—to the day—I lost him. When it became necessary that I go through his personal belongings, I found my letter carefully placed in a zip-lock plastic bag in his personal file.

No one will ever know how many times I've thanked God that I wrote that letter. Writing it has taught me to let anyone I care about know how I feel *now*. I don't wait. Tomorrow may be too late.

Following are the jingles and sentiment printed on the commercial Happy Anniversary card in which I enclosed my letter and a copy of the letter itself.

> To the Guy who
> knows me like a book
>
> and somehow eats
> the things I cook
>
> who puts up with
> my every whim
>
> and makes up
> when I'm mad at him
>
> who's seen me when
> I'm not a beauty
>
> the Guy who helps
> with household duty
>
> who knows when
> I exceed my budget
>
> but who's too thoughtful
> to begrudge it.

my Helpmate
my Partner
and Breadwinner

The man who takes
me out to dinner (hint)

The one I depend on,
in bright or stormy weather!
Sure glad we took
That plunge together
Happy Anniversary
with all my love

                    Wanda

                To Morgan

11/26/37   11/26/77

It was November 26, 1937 . . . just 40 years ago today. Remember the little white-haired minister who thought Frank R. was the about-to-be bridegroom? Frank was the nervous one. You were as cool as though getting married was an everyday happening. But then, you always kept your cool, and still do, where things that matter are concerned.

Remember that overcast November day, the Lake of the Ozarks, the small sinking fishing boat and you rowing four of us to safety. I remember it vividly. Bob G. was too scared to help, and Lavergne and I too inept to spell you at the oars. You knew, perhaps Bob did, too, but it wasn't until later that I learned we were over 90 feet of water when the boat started to sink.

Water always held a certain fascination for you. Through you I learned to enjoy it, although there was always a small, haunting fear when we were in open water. I often think of your admonition to me, "Don't be afraid of water, but have great respect for it."

Remember the fun-filled weekends at Willoughby-On-The-Lake? and the time you grabbed me by the seat of my swimsuit when the undertow of a huge Erie wave sent me "ass over teakettle" as you so graphically related my up-ended position to friends?

And remember the fun we had with our first little boat? The small aluminum fishing boat? I never caught many fish. I was too busy snagging a tree limb, an underwater stump or hooking the seat of my pants. But, you never seemed to mind re-baiting my hook or extricating me from fouled-up lines.

And our first cruiser? Remember how proud we were? You had worked all winter on it . . . cleaning, scraping, painting. My contribution was to re-dye the canvas seat covers. It was many days and much scrubbing before my hands lost their aqua tinge. Oh, and our first long boat trip? To see Fred and Lelia in Chicago? Our first day out, remember we tied up alongside an old grain barge and caught so many channel cats we had to throw most of them back? And later, crossing Peoria Lake, how we, rather how *you*, rode out the tail end of a tornado. All I could do was peer through the darkness to try to help you stay in the channel. And out on Lake Michigan, remember how you and Fred laughed when I hid my head under a pillow in the cabin, while the two of you had a ball heading into what I thought were gigantic waves?

And speaking of Chicago. . . . Remember how you "sky-jacked" me on our 15th anniversary? It was a fabulous weekend. You had planned everything . . . down to the last detail . . . even to my toothbrush and pajamas . . . and adjoining rooms at the Stevens for Fred and Lelia as our guests.

So many, many wonderful memories . . . holding hands and dreaming in front of the library fire at Mother and Dad's . . . deep sea fishing off the Kona Coast . . . cruising to Block Island with Sturg . . . buying fresh swordfish at Point Judith . . . quohogging on the Cape . . .

But all the memories are not of seagoing yachts or walking barefoot on the moonlit beach at Waikiki, or going to sleep lulled by the surf and the soft strumming of guitars . . . or eating oysters at Felix's . . . or the excitement of watching a Kentucky Derby and drinking mint juleps at the Pendennis Club . . . or paddle-wheeling down the Mississippi on the old "Golden Eagle."

No, some of our memories are sad . . . some still hurt. But those, too, we shared . . . and still share. There was the fire at Echo Valley and the loss of our loved little "wires" . . . our disappointment in Bob . . . the heartache when we read Fritzi's letter telling us about Fred and Lelia . . . Bea's and later Lou's untimely death.

And, as in any marriage of two strong people, we've had our disagreements and the angry words, we've both wished we'd never uttered. Somehow the angry words, like the hurtful memories, have been only a vague and distant counterpoint to the happy memories, making the latter stand out in bold relief.

Yes, so many memories! How could we ever forget "Puddle's" little family and your call to me in Lisbon (in the wee small hours) to tell me of the event . . . or our missed connections in Madrid (we laugh now, but it wasn't funny at the time) . . . or how proud I was when you were chosen to handle that special assignment in Kuwait for Getty Oil . . . or how pleased you were when I was made SBF's and St. Louis' first woman merchandise manager . . . or the day we bought PUDGY II and later our tandem trip to Kentucky Lake with the Hedenkamps . . . or that never-to-be-forgotten week in San Francisco, staying at the Mark and dancing to the music of Bob Wellman . . . or our many trips to New Orleans and the Sugar Bowl games . . . Doug and Beulah . . . "Billy" and Art . . . Ralph and Louise and the small 25 pounds of ice . . . Carnival in Havana . . . that long ago meeting in Steubenville to get our marriage license . . . and our first "home," that apartment in Pittsburgh? Remember Liz and Tommy Kincheloe, the Steeles, Steins and the other young couples in the building? We were all so young and so very broke. Remember how we took turns each Saturday night playing host and hostess? With each couple kicking in for the food and beer?

And will you ever forget our Dutchman, Anton? Or your phone call to him and his "tomato" in Germany? Or Skyline Drive after a sleet storm . . . or the summer house you built? And the lazy summer evenings we spent in it. Or the swaying 30 foot ladder and the flying squirrels? What a magnificent montage our memories make. Winter nights at Echo Valley when the snow fell softly and we listened to music and watched the embers burn low . . . summer days on a Mississippi sandbar (remember when Fella II swam the width of that wide river? I silently cry whenever I think of the love and courage he displayed when he thought we had left him).

There are so many heartfelt memories it's hard to recall when each happened . . . in what spring . . . or which December. . . .

I do know that these I've mentioned are but a few of those engraved in my heart.

There are the songs that have special significance . . . Russ Morgan's "Does Your Heart Beat for Me?" and "Careless" to name a couple . . . and the imaginative gifts you always gave me . . . like the bouquet of roses tied with a huge bow of dollars bills (you had laboriously scotch-taped, end to end, 100 new one dollar bills to make a long tyable ribbon).

Even our "Little People" from our first "Fella," who'd tackle anything if it were bigger than he . . . little "Frosty" who died in your arms of a heart attack . . . to "Petie," "Spunky," "Fella II," "Buttons," "Puddles," "Muffin," . . . even "Missy" (who took the seat out of "Pop" Wedelick's pants) and all the little waifs we took in along the way. They gave us love, loyalty and so much pleasure. They, too, are part of the memories that have given rich meaning to 40 treasured and unforgettable years.

There's a short poem I once read that says it all far better than I:

> There'll always be a pathway
> where we'll stroll hand in hand
> There'll always be a hilltop
> where alone we two may stand.
> There'll always be a trysting place
> where we two never part . . .
> a sacred shrine of memories
> Down deep within my heart.
>
> With Love
> Wanda

God willing, we'll continue . . . hand in hand, with our making of memories.

May 6, 1985

If I were Jewish or if my life or that of any of my loved ones had ever been threatened, I'm certain it would be very difficult for me to say or even if I could say, "I think it's time we softpeddle the Bittburg issue."

But I'm not Jewish, I've never been threatened, I've never been in military service. It may be I'm lacking in empathy and just don't understand, but somehow or other I feel protestors and media alike have wrung the subject dry—harangued it to the point where many people think, regardless of their sympathies, the repetitious comments not only have opened old wounds but have salted them.

May 8, 1985

By choice, today started very early for me. I turned my TV on at 6:00 A.M. to catch NBC's "Sunrise News." I wanted to hear President Reagan's entire address (boos and all) before the European Parliament in Strasbourg, France.

Often on later telecasts of important events only excerpts are shown. Like "Ralph, who ate the whole thing," I wanted to listen to the whole thing. I wanted to evaluate Mr. Regan's words and digest them without the benefit of media opinion.

I was misty-eyed when Mr. Reagan finished and, as I so often am, was proud to be an American—proud, too, that Mr. Reagan expressed so well my innermost feelings and philosophy.

I've often wondered why this president always touched a responsive chord in me. It isn't his shiny black hair or his ability to chop wood. (Morgan could do it better and looked more graceful.) It's his philosophy of government, his belief that if given the opportunity, man takes pride in doing for himself. Basically, man doesn't want a handout even if it's the easy way out. I believe Mr. Reagan appeals to the dignity that resides—or should reside—in each of us.

May 9, 1985

A day on the town—well, hardly, but a visit to the opthamologist, the dentist, and luncheon away from the nursing home plus a very satisfactory therapy workout upon my return, made it an enjoyable, exhilarating day.

Mrs. Bono, COTG director, was kind enough to take me and a COTG nurse aide to assist me on my round of appointments. It was my pleasure to take both Mrs. Bono and the aide to luncheon.

The women's exchange being in the same building as my dentist, we settled for luncheon there, amidst the chattering and laughter of two or three dozen females, exchanging pleasantries—a typical "ladies' tea-room" atmosphere. The food, as always, was delicious.

We left the nursing home at 9:00 A.M. and returned at 3:00 P.M.—a long, tiring day for me in my wheelchair, but a very happy day, nevertheless.

May 10, 1985

I'm seventy-seven years old today—a good time for me to bow my head in gratitude for all the blessings that have come my way.

Today turned out to be one of my happiest. Both weather-wise and friendship-wise, it was beautiful. There were many phone calls, both local and long-distance, flowers, and small gifts.

Meredith P—— called from Princeton, New Jersey. Bonnie and Jim Ream wired flowers from Florida, my dear friend Emily B—— sent a lovely arrangement of spring flowers, and many of my former buyers sent or called greetings.

My little third-grader, my pen pal, Michelle Backes, not only brought me a birthday card she had made and a lovely potted plant, she brought her mother, dad, older sister, and little brother to see me. They are a delightful family, and I thoroughly enjoyed meeting them.

Another highlight—one of our former COTG aides, Linda Gearhart, a woman I admire very much, brought her daughter to meet me. The daughter, Beth, is entering college this fall. I was flattered that this lovely young girl wanted to meet me.

I'm going to bed now with Eve and Ken Wilde's gift, the autobiography of Lee Iacocca. I know I'm going to love this book, because this man's accomplishments or what I know about them have seemed to me to be an expression of the American Dream or what made this country great.

Tonight "my cup [truly] runneth over."

May 12, 1985

Mother's Day

The nurse aide asked me what *my* mother was like. How do I describe a small (five-foot-two) energetic bundle of love, talent, personality, and charm—except to say my father and I thought she was someone very special.

She was an accomplished pianist and could play anything either by note or by ear. There were many evenings when Dad and I (often, friends, too) sat listening to her play—it might be classical, it might be ragtime, or it might be something she'd improvised. On occasion, my father would join in with his violin, which he said he played for his own "amazement." Mother, of course, thought he was another Heifetz.

My parents were married sixty-four years before my mother's too-big-for-her-body heart gave out.

She was the stabilizing, as well as the motivating, influence among her many friends and especially my father and me, who adored her.

Imagine! My social calendar has been so full I haven't had the opportunity to write in my journal for a couple of days. (Honest, I'm not being facetious.)

The COTG mother/daughter dinner Tuesday evening, May 14, was beautifully handled and very heartwarming. Emily B—— came as my daughter/guest. Even though she is in the midst of moving to her new home, she managed to find time for me. Friends with birthday greetings are still stopping by or calling, and belated floral greetings are still arriving. One of the loveliest was from Ida and Charles Grissom, who have never forgotten me on my birthday. Charlie was one of Morgan's friends of long standing.

I've decided that being seventy-seven isn't half bad. In fact, being over three-quarters of a century old has turned out to be like vintage wine. If properly aged and decanted, it is mellow, satisfying, and often appreciated.

How glad I am that I haven't turned to vinegar, as so often happens with wine and people. And how did that come about? I believe that like starting with good grapes, my genes were also good. Add to that my disciplined and Christian upbringing during my formative years and my education, both academic and through experience; all that has contributed to my ability to come to terms with my life, even during its upheavals, and to accept with relative composure and equanimity whatever comes my way.

I've reached the point where I can sincerely repeat, "I'm as contented and happy as I can be without Morgan and without living in a home of my own."

It was difficult for me to put the book down, but I've just finished reading Lee Iacocca's autobiography. I admired him even more now than I did during the Chrysler travail.

If possible, his story strengthened my beliefs in the free enterprise system and in the ultimate success of any individual who sets goals and tries hard enough. Only one or two Iacocca's comments bothered me a bit—and that I dismissed because I'm such a die-hard Reaganite. After Iacocca made several TV commercials, he was rumored as a possible presidential candidate. His reply to that was, "I guess this rumor started because of all the TV commercials I made for Chrysler.

Many people now think I'm an actor. Everybody knows being an actor doesn't quality you to be president.''

I thought that snide remark was beneath him—particularly in the light of all the personal hurts he'd endured. I thought, too, it negated much of his rhetoric regarding his understanding and empathy for the other guy.

I did like his comments regarding labor's demands for fringe benefits, the cost of living allowance (COLA), and the thirty-and-out regulation espoused by management. I probably liked those comments because I agreed with them. For what it is worth, I thought his biography objectively written for the most part with only an occasional bias showing through.

I particularly felt his urging management, labor, and government to get together not only timely but necessary if we are to preserve the American Dream.

I sincerely hope this book is widely read. It's time Americans started working as a team.

May 18, 1985

Yesterday while looking for some information asked for by COTG's activity director, I finally found the packet of letters and cards I've been searching for for months.

Today I've been on a sentimental journey, rereading those letters and cards written and sent to me by Morgan before and during our marriage. Some of the letters were written to me while he was on business trips; many of his letters were lost in the fire at Echo Valley.

Included in the packet were a couple of notes and bits of free verse written by me and inserted in the packet when I asked to have it filed.

Although many of his letters were lost in the fire, I found enough yesterday to let me say, as Anna did in *The King and I,* "I had a love of my own."

That love was and is enough to sustain me the rest of my life. One of my inserted notes, dated April 26, 1978, said: "The Beginning and The End . . .''

Notes and mementoes from the in-between years were mostly lost in the Echo Valley Farm fire of November 22, 1970.

"Wanda and Morgan were married November 26, 1937. Morgan and most of Wanda died February 26, 1978.''

Among the too-numerous to mention things I don't understand
are:

1. The *reasoning* of those people who complain about the
   economy, the unavailability of "good jobs," their difficulty
   in meeting expenses and paying bills, yet don't show up for
   work on the job they have or call in saying they don't feel
   up to par and doesn't one's health come first? Of course,
   there are times when the illness "excuse" is legitimate. But
   there are many times, too, when it's simply an excuse. I've
   worked all my life—a short time as a social worker, longer
   as a newspaper woman, and even longer as a retail buyer
   and executive. I know that in all of those working years,
   forty-five to be exact, there were many mornings when I
   would have preferred to stay in bed, laze in the sun, or go
   on an outing with friends. I didn't—probably because of the
   combination of genes and discipline I mentioned earlier.
2. What *happened* to "a job well done?" "Good enough" is
   a phrase still too much in use today.
3. *Why* are so many women discontented, even unhappy,
   about being women? I believe all my life I've agreed with
   the song "I Enjoy Being a Girl." I always loved using fragrance, wearing high-heeled shoes, sheer hosiery, and pretty
   undies, and knowing how to wear a scarf to dress up a
   costume, yes, and taking care of my home (in addition to
   working and traveling). I was always so proud when I entertained and our friends complimented me on our home
   and the food I served. Morgan, of course, was the smart one.
   He praised me as a hostess, for my dinner parties, and for
   my ability to handle a large party. As a result, I knocked
   myself out trying to please him. In other words, I've loved
   being a woman.

I just read in the *Monitor* that May 15 marked the thirtieth anniversary of the unification of Austria.

My first visit to Austria was in 1953, when four-power rule was
still the order of the day. The U.S.A., Great Britain, the USSR, and

France exchanged authority every thirty days. The Soviets were in power when I arrived at Schwechat Airport on a flight from Zurich to Vienna.

My seat companion on that flight was a gentleman by the name (if I remember correctly) of Rudolf Sills, director of Programs and Operations for the U.S.–controlled Red-White-Red network in Vienna. We chatted for some time, and when Mr. Sills found out that I was a fashion jewelry buyer (my job at the time), he asked if I planned to go into upper Austria to see the Czech jewelry makers . . . the refugees who were making their way from under the Iron Curtain into Linz and the small towns along the road to Wels.

I knew that Gablonz or Jablonec, Czechoslovakia, had been a jewelry center, that the Sudetenland Germans controlled the industry, and that the Czechs had turned against the Germans and were making their way one by one into West Germany, particularly into that area around Kaufbeuren. I wasn't aware of any settlement in upper Austria. I was intrigued, however, and when Mr. Sills gave me the name of a Dr. Leopold Unger, director of Caritas, the charitable organization that was looking after the needs of the refugees, I decided then to visit Linz.

This would take a bit of doing, however, as my itinerary only called for one working day in Vienna. Any change of plan would necessarily alter my plane and hotel reservations and working appointments and, in general, create no end of trouble, not only for me but for the foreign offices with which I was working. I decided I'd go and play it by ear.

Mr. Sills helped me through Austrian customs and to the antiquated airport bus (held together by baling wire, string, chewing gum, and faith). The bus hiccoughed its way to the Vienna terminal via the only highway the Soviets permitted us to use. Any deviation was cause for arrest, as was any deviation from prescribed areas in Vienna proper, Mr. Sills explained.

I was met at the terminal in Vienna by the head of our Austrian buying office, a short, affable Viennese, a Mr. Kornbichler, who was to act as my interpreter and guide. When I asked him about the jewelry-making refugees, he said that he'd heard some were settling in the Linz area, but since he hadn't worked with any jewelry buyers since the war's end and since the Vienna office had only recently reopened, he frankly hadn't done any research . . . however, if I wanted to make the trip and if my papers were in order, he'd gladly go with me. It was then about 5: 00 P.M., and we would have time to catch the Orient Express, which would get us to Linz about midnight. The Orient Express then operating was an international train plying between Bucharest and Paris, and Herr Kornbichler felt there would be no "incidents."

After hurriedly contacting Dr. Unger, who gave me the names of the Czech jewelry makers, living in the various little towns around Linz and Wels, I checked into the old Hotel Sacher and quickly repacked my flight bag. I recall taking time to touch the silk-damask–covered walls of my room and the matching lounge chairs and stare at the huge Bohemian crystal chandelier that hung from the center of the ceiling. It was all breathtakingly "Old World," I thought, and I could almost visualize Anna Sacher strolling the corridors smoking a big, black cigar (as history tells us) and arranging a rendezvous for one of Franz Josef's court. I made many later trips to Vienna and at one time or other stopped at all the better hotels in that ancient city, but no hotel room ever left the impression as did that first, baronial, unremodeled room at the Sacher.

The ride to Linz was uneventful. The train passed alongside the Vienna woods and the Danube. Try as I did, with my face pressed against the window, I couldn't see much because of the darkness. (I made up for that on later trips by driving the distance and loving every storybook village along the way.)

About midnight the train pulled onto the Enns Bridge over the Enns River and came to a halt midstream. This, I learned from Herr Kornbichler, was the dividing line between the American and the Soviet zones. Within minutes, Soviet soldiers mounted the train. Two young uniformed Russians, who couldn't have been more than sixteen or seventeen years of age, came to my compartment, where "Little Hanns" (as I later came to call him) and I sat talking.

One soldier stood at my compartment door with his arms akimbo. The other stepped forward and held out his hand for my passport and papers. I looked up and smiled. There was no response . . . not a change of expression on either of the two young, sullen faces. The one soldier took my passport, visas, and the all-important gray card, which had permitted my entrance into the Soviet Zone. The lad very carefully read my passport upside-down until he came to my picture, which was then upside-down, too. He quickly turned the passport around and glanced to see if I had noticed. I pretended I hadn't. An hour and a half later, the soldiers dismounted and the train pulled across the center of the bridge into the American Zone and a deserted, blacked-out Linz.

At that hour there were no cabs at the railroad station. There was, however, one sleepy attendant who gave Herr Kornbichler and me some vague, arm-waving directions. Little Hanns and I started to walk. We eventually found our way in the darkness to the newly opened Hotel Park, a Marshall Plan venture. We checked in and made arrangements to have a car and driver pick us up the next morning at 8: 00 A.M. I remember it was a very short night!

The next day I located and worked with some twenty refugee families who were living and working in abandoned German army barracks and horse stables. Even now I can feel the numbing cold of those buildings, where whole families worked, cooked, and slept in a space not much larger than a narrow one-car garage. I still remember one barracks home in particular, perhaps because it seemed warmer than the other bone-chilling rooms I'd entered. I unbuttoned my coat and removed my gloves . . . something I hadn't been warm enough to do in the other homes. I remember being settled at a workbench, discussing quality requirements with this home manufacturer, when I felt something warm snuggle up against my ankle. I looked down and saw a puppy curled up at my feet. I remember thinking, *How nice that kids and dogs always seemed to like me.*

I wasn't so smug later when I found upon leaving that the puppy had gummed a good pair of silk-lined kid gloves into a soggy mess. As for the little towns between Linz and Wels, I believe their names will always remain with me . . . Linz, Enns, Krems, Kremsmunster, Steyr, Steyr-Klenck, Stey-Munichholz, and finally Wels, where Herr Kornbichler and I dismissed our car and driver and caught the 7: 15 P.M. Arlberg Express back to Vienna and, for me, the Hotel Sacher. It had been a long, exhausting twenty-four hours, but I had kept to my itinerary and caught my scheduled flight back to Paris the next day.

I don't think I ever worked as hard—or accomplished as much—as I did in those twenty-four hours. I was told later that my efforts helped a great deal in opening the Austrian jewelry market in America. I'll always be glad about that.

May 22, 1985

The Miss Kitty Dancers from Six Flags entertained COTG residents last evening. Our dining room was transformed into an Old West saloon, with the department heads dressed as dance hall girls and the dietary staff, waiters, and waitresses wearing the garb of cowgirls, cowboys, and ranch hands. Soft drinks, beer, pretzels, and potato chips were served at a bar and available at the tables.

Today some of the residents were talking about the fun evening—how attractive our dance hall girls were, about gamblers, gaming tables, et cetera. Someone mentioned the phrase "lucky seven." I replied, "If seven is lucky, then I'm double-lucky, because I'm seventy-seven." The reply to that was, "How can you say that you're that lucky when most of your life is over?" Perhaps "the best is yet to be." I don't know, I only know I'm not fearful of the future.

Perhaps my composure regarding the future is predicated upon my belief that my body is only the mortal shell housing that spirit or God/power-given life that is within each of us. I like to think that when my body gives out, the spirit (some call it energy) is released and joins or becomes part of that all prevailing, vast, uncharted Universal Energy. To me that might be the eternal life referred to in the Bible—or it might be a kind of reincarnation, in which many people believe.

I can't help but wonder, if there is a transference of energy, could that be the "conservation of energy" to which some folks refer? There are so many imponderables, and I'm certainly no metaphysicist. Only my faith tells me there's no cause for apprehension.

All because someone mentioned "lucky seven," I went off on this pseudo-metaphysical tangent.

May 23, 1985

Yesterday a group of us spent most of the day as guests of Highcroft Ridge School. What a joy those youngsters are! Every hour of the day was memorable, from the large sign and waiting students in front of the building welcoming COTG to the entertainment and delicious fried chicken luncheon.

I was so pleased when three of my previous pen pals made it a point to find me and say hello. We toured the classrooms, watched exercises in the gym, joined the craftmaking, and admired the student craftwork on display in the corridors. The entertainment was good and I'm sure represented hours of practice. The third-graders sang "We Are the World." The sixth-graders presented a musical version of Tom Sawyer and his friends whitewashing Aunt Polly's fence. Everyone from Mr. Overfelt, the principal, to the teachers and smallest kindergartner made us oldsters feel welcome and wanted.

May 24, 1985

Nine of us were invited by Mrs. Bono to have luncheon at her home today. The luncheon was super and was prepared almost entirely by our hostess. Several days ago, I sent my wheelchair back to the dealer for a "tune-up." It was to take two or three days. In the interim, I was given a loaner to use. My "chariot" had a right-hand drive to compensate for my useless left hand. The loaner, a real clunker, requiring two hands to operate efficiently, left me exhausted by day's end just trying to keep from "driving" in circles.

When the dealer returned my chair yesterday, I was delighted, and after paying him $160.00 for the work done, I started off down the corridor, pleased that I was in my own vehicle again. I hadn't gone very far when Doris stopped me, asking when I was going to return her chair. I explained that I had just had this chair overhauled and that it really was my chair.

"The hell it is," she answered. With that, she approached another wheelchair resident. One way or another, I thought, she was going to locate a chair. She often appropriates a wheelchair in which she can cruise around the halls.

The nurses kindly dispossess her and return the wheelchair to its rightful owner. This happens quite regularly, as Doris enjoys her wheelchair cruising or joy-riding, as one of the residents calls it.

May 26, 1986

Yesterday Mickie F. and I listened to (Mickie is blind) and watched William Buckley's "Firing Line" program. A philosophical discussion regarding the difference between contentment and happiness was in progress when we turned in on the program.

Prof. Mortimer Adler of the Chicago Philosophical Research Institute was saying that contentment was a matter of attitude but that happiness was a matter of morality.

I listened carefully to his reasoning, agreed with him where contentment was concerned, but thought the definition of happiness should be enlarged upon.

I think that happiness is a spiritual quality or feeling like love or peace of mind or tranquillity. I believe, too, happiness can be achieved if one is willing to work for it. Marriage, for example, can bring about happiness if the two people involved are willing to forget self long enough to consider the other person's feelings, attitudes, and opinions.

Adjustments and compromise on the part of each person can, more often than not, create a climate conducive to that feeling I call "happiness." I wonder if that concern for the other person's feelings is what Adler considers morality. If so, I agree.

May 27, 1985

When residents are cross and grumpy or complaining, refuse to take their medicine, or are in general balky, the aides say, "It's a full moon tonight." Last evening one of the aides came to my room and asked if the moon was full. I told her that I didn't know but that we could check a calendar I had in my desk. It would indicate the state of the moon. She said, "Never mind. I know it has to be a full moon tonight. I've just spent the last thirty minutes helping a maintenance man retrieve the blouse Marie B—— flushed down the toilet."

May 29, 1985

Arthur B. Baer frequently said facetiously, "Now, if I owned this business, I'd . . ." Then he'd go on to say what he'd do or wouldn't do. More often than not, his ideas were adopted or expanded or became the nucleus of later action by his two partners at SBF.

I'm certainly not even a partner in any nursing home business (and it is a business), but if I were, there's definitely one thing I would *not* do. I would *not oversell* the facility's capability of providing therapy or restorative aide assistance unless there was sufficient staff to back up those claims or promises.

May 30, 1985

Shades of my retailing past . . . I'm very annoyed by the way basic stocks are reordered or *not* reordered by the COTG dietary department.

COTG has been in and out of certain fruit juices for almost two weeks. Residents are grousing and one resident in particular says her doctor prescribed cranberry juice for her and she hasn't had any for a week. Someone—whoever is responsible for ordering food supplies—is careless or lazy, as I see no excuse for being out of something as basic as "sugar in a grocery store." I'm sure most department store employees are familiar with that expression.

May 31, 1985

I'm grumpy and my last entry shows it. Guess it's time I did a bit of serious talking to me. Changing the direction of my thinking might put me in a better mood.

I'll try tax reform, as that's about all I've heard on TV or radio the last few days. If I recall correctly, several presidents have tried their hands at tax reforms but the U.S. still has a tax code that consists of one thousand pages of incomprehensible jargon.

I read an article not too long ago in which an Edward R. Kantowicz (I hope I spelled his name correctly) was quoted as saying, "Attempts to reform cash management, taxation, health, or welfare are doomed unless they are bold and comprehensive."

I've heard others, whose opinions I respect, say piecemeal efforts are futile and that only a full-scale offensive will succeed. That makes sense to me. Piecemeal attempts can be plea-bargained away. Lobbyists and self-serving politicians step in with counterproposals that destroy the total reform effort. Look what happened to Carter's three-martini luncheon cuts. Nothing! Whittling away is hardly worth the effort, I believe.

Reagan's plan to me seems bold and comprehensive. I hope there will be enough bipartisan and compromise support to effect a tax plan that is simpler and more fair than that which we struggle with now.

June 1, 1985

They were in the TV room, quarreling as usual. Joe wanted to watch a baseball game. Annie wanted to watch anything but a baseball game. They had been switching channels back and forth for at least fifteen minutes. Finally, in exasperation, Joe shouted, "Annie, leave the room!" Smiling sweetly, Annie replied, "I'll be glad to, Joe. Just tell me where you want me to leave it."

June 3, 1985

The new resident with the German sounding name asked me if there were many foreigners in this nursing home. I replied that as far as I knew there weren't any. "You're mistaken," she answered. Pointing to a woman a few feet away, she continued, "Just listen to her!" I turned my head and recognized a German born resident who had lived in this country many years, was a naturalized citizen, and had raised her family here. I explained all that, ending with, "She just hasn't lost her German accent."

I should have left it at that. Instead, I went on to say I didn't think her German name and accent made her a foreigner. Still not knowing when to leave things alone, I called attention to our names, both of which were of German origin. The new resident then said, "That's different. I'm an American; besides, she talks funny."

My explanation that the only native born Americans were the American Indians and that all the rest of us had foreign blood in us to one extent or another only left her with an expression of incredulity on her face. I couldn't help thinking that oldsters certainly aren't immune from bigotry and it doesn't stop at nursing home doors. Too, I wondered if the new resident thought I was something from outer space or just all "Greek"?

June 4, 1985

Several months ago I was seriously thinking about buying a computer, with the idea of taking a college course or two—perhaps a refresher course in psychology, philosophy, math, or government—anything to keep me busy and thinking (my prescription for being alone and not becoming lonely).

I even went so far as to contact the California based Electronic University to find out what courses were available and what make computers were compatible with their software. My friends, when they heard of my interest, began sending me computer magazines, books, and articles regarding computers. I'm swamped!

June 26, 1985

I see in *Construction News and Review* that St. Louis Union Station, which has been undergoing renovation since 1983, will be ready for public viewing as a festive marketplace on August 29. I understand there will be a spectacular opening ceremony.

I have no desire to attend the opening ceremony, but I'd like so much to visit the renovated station sometime afterward. That magnificent old building fascinates me for three reasons:

1. Its history has intrigued me ever since I came to St. Louis in 1940.
2. Morgan always felt St. Louis should do something with the building and site in the way of restoration. He was one of the station's boosters even during its declining years. How pleased he would be to know what has been done.
3. Some forty years ago Union Station was the starting point for all of my buying trips. They were usually to New York via the New York Central and the Pennsylvania Railroads. I could go on a nostalgic binge now just thinking about those trips and the people I knew and worked with then.

Regarding the station's history, it was completed in 1894. Since then its 230-foot clock tower and facade of immense Bedford limestone have held a special place in the hearts of many St. Louisans.

The station, the grandest of Grand Union stations, larger than New York's Grand Central, was designed by St. Louis architect Theodore C. Link, winner in 1891 of a national competition sponsored by the Terminal Railroad Association to design what was conceived as the country's largest railway terminal. It took three years to build at a cost of $6.5 million. The renovation, costing $135 million, is considered to be one of the country's largest renovation attempts.

According to *Construction News*: "It's the most exciting project to hit St. Louis since an enigmatic over-sized wicket was planted on the 'Gateway of the West' River Bank 25 years ago."

The Rouse Company of Columbia, Maryland, the developer, also developed such marketplaces as Faneuil Hall in Boston, Harbor Place in Baltimore, and The Gallery in Philadelphia.

There's so much to be told about this old building and yards—its size, et cetera, and what the renovation will bring. The train shed is still the largest single span train shed in the world (twice the size of Grand Central's). At the turn of the century when it was built, it drew international attention.

I understand the total site covers some 60 acres . . . 11.5 acres enclosed within the world-renowned shed. The renovation will include a luxury hotel with restaurants, a 162,000 square foot space for retail shops, a one-acre lake, an amphitheater, parking for two thousand cars . . . to name just a few of the features. It was in 1978 that the last train pulled out of the shed.

How proud St. Louis must be today of the grand old station!

June 27, 1985

I watched Yul Brynner being interviewed on TV this morning. He said he was retiring from *The King and I* . . . after some forty-five hundred performances. I've seen him several times as the king since his opening on Broadway, but I'm glad I had the opportunity to first see him with Gertrude Lawrence and the original cast. To me, Lawrence was the unforgettable Anna.

June 28, 1985

Turning my thoughts to Siam, I recall my first trip there in the early sixties. It was 1961, to be exact. Of course, it was called Thailand by then. Although Bangkok's newly built Erwan was suggested, I chose to stop at the Oriental Hotel.

A large skylight in the Oriental lobby permitted sunlight or moonlight to silhouette the small tropical garden below. The floors were all teakwood, as was the wide stairway that led to the upper levels. My room was on a wing with windows overlooking the outdoor tropical garden and the Chao Phraya (river).

The floor of my room was covered with a rug of straw matting. An antiquated air-conditioner groaned in one of the windows, and a "flit" gun filled with insect spray lay near a container of fresh flowers on a bedside table.

A pull chain commode and a clean but vintage tub were highlights of the small bathroom.

My first impression was that I was encountering some locale from Maugham's "Rain."

I was almost convinced of it when the young Thai lad who brought my luggage to me asked if I was comfortable, then queried, "Gentleman?" I replied, "No, my husband isn't here, and thank you, I'm quite comfortable." It wasn't until three sentences later that I realized that he meant did I want a gentleman. I emphasized that I did not. He smiled and nodded to indicate he understood.

I didn't see or hear from him again until morning, when he

knocked on my door to announce the time. I was thus awakened every morning with a gentle knock on the door and a whispered "Time to get up."

Although the Oriental had been renovated and modernized, on subsequent trips I stopped at the Dusit Thani. However, on each trip I tried to have dinner at least once during my stay in Bangkok in the outdoor garden of the Oriental, where the water of the Chao Phraya softly lapped at the piling and boat dock at the garden's edge.

I'd always been glad I had the experience of stopping at the Oriental, when it was reminiscent of all I'd ever visualized about the South Seas or a tropical land.

I still find the old hotel, as it once was, had charm and atmosphere, if nothing else.

June 29, 1985

The new resident was small, attractive, and intelligent, but had an aura of sadness about her. I thought that she was too young to find it necessary to live in a nursing home.

Although she never said in so many words, from what she did tell me, I could only guess that her husband hadn't been able to come to terms with her disability, which is a severe one.

She has managed to accept her physical condition, but hasn't come to terms with her husband's lack of understanding. At times, they appear so close to bridging the gap—but mentally so far from actually doing it.

I wonder how many couples have similar problems. Probably more than we realize.

June 30, 1985

Several of us were sitting on the patio, sunning ourselves and chatting. Someone mentioned age. One oldster said he was an old man and that he hated it. A woman seated nearby said she knew just how he felt . . . that living was nothing more than day-to-day existence and that she'd be glad when the end came.

Another woman spoke up, saying she didn't want to die but she didn't want to go on living like this either. Nothing was like it once was, she continued.

The first old gentleman interrupted, "But you're lucky. Your children come to see you and take you out on occasion. Mine don't even know I exist."

"Yes," the woman answered, "they come to see me, but only to lecture me. You'd think I didn't have a brain in my head. I don't know how I, being so mentally retarded, was able to produce and raise such smart kids. They don't understand why I don't like it here. Wouldn't you think they'd see that this place is nothing like my home? They keep asking why I don't enter into more of the activities . . . why I don't get interested in something." Going on and on, she said, "What is there to get interested in around here? That garrulous old man in the room next to mine? No, thank you. As my grandson would say, 'I'm bored out of my skull.' "

I listened for a while, thinking, *They haven't learned to accept change. The sooner they learn, the happier they'll be. . . . At least they'll be more content.*

They don't realize we live in a world of changes. Life itself is activity and growth. None of us can keep things as they were or even as they are now. "Things come to pass. Nothing can last."

At ninety years old, my father was the youngest person, in attitude, that I've ever known. He believed that no one grows old *but that when one stopped growing and learning he was old.*

How wise he was and how pleased I am that some of his philosophy rubbed off on me. I know I can meet change . . . not always calmly . . . but confidently, because I've learned (often the hard way) that with every change and new experience I am growing.

July 1, 1985

I had such a pleasant surprise yesterday. Michelle Backes, my little pen pal the third-grader, called to ask if she and her family might stop by to see me. She explained that her grandparents and an aunt from out of town were visiting and she'd like for me to meet them. Of course, I said yes.

A short time later they arrived, and what a lovely family they are! There were Mom, Dad, and older sister Jennifer and little brother Michael, all of whom Michelle had brought to see me once before. This time, the grandparents and aunt were added. They were equally charming. I thoroughly enjoyed their visit!

July 2, 1985

I didn't know whether to be amused, embarrassed, angry, frightened, or concerned. On second thought, I think I was 50 percent amused, 50 percent embarrassed, and only slightly annoyed and concerned.

I was *amused* because I must have looked like an aging stripteaser last evening. I was as naked as the cliched jaybird, seated in the lowered whirlpool chair at the bottom of the deep whirlpool tub. I had just finished my whirlpool bath and was prepared to be lifted mechanically from the tub when the mechanism refused to function.

The aide who attended me, seeing the chair wouldn't rise, emptied the tub of water, draped a couple of bath towels around my shoulders, called for help, and before I could say "why me?" I was surrounded by two RNs who didn't know what to do and several aides who were exchanging ideas as to how to get me out of my tub without breaking my leg, foot, or neck. I asked only that none attempt to lift me who didn't know how to manipulate the muscles of my paralyzed leg.

Finally, the aide who had helped rescue me the other time the chair had gone balky with me in it suggested that a gait belt be put on me so that there would be something to hang onto besides my wet body.

I was soon lifted out of the deep tub, ensconced in a robe, taken to my room, and put to bed. I was *embarrassed* because again my privacy had been invaded, necessarily this time. The other time the mechanism refused to lower the chair, I was left suspended in the air, feet dangling, while I alternately looked at the ceiling and watched the aides below trying to figure out how to get me out of the chair and into the water without hurting me. The feat was accomplished that time, too.

Considering that I've taken a whirlpool bath every night since I've been at COTG, I don't feel I have much room for complaint, annoyance, or concern.

July 3, 1985

Writing of experiences as I did a few entries back, I'm reminded of another experience I had in Bangkok on my first trip.

The office of the commissionaire with whom I worked in Bangkok was a branch of its larger Hong Kong office. There were six very intelligent young Chinese lads in the Thai office who, during my stay in Bangkok, assisted me. The day before I left Thailand for New Delhi, the boys decided they'd take me to luncheon. Knowing I liked Chinese cuisine, they selected a small restaurant known for Shanghaiese cooking.

Whenever and wherever I traveled, I always tried to learn something about each country's food, and I often said, "If the food is clean, fresh, and nonpoisonous, I'll try it." That particular time I almost didn't even try it.

When the boat that took the seven of us (the six lads and me) down the *klong* (canal) pulled up at the restaurant boat dock, I noted how clean and freshly scrubbed everything was. Then when we each selected a live fish from the water tank, I knew the fish we wanted prepared were fresh. I then assumed the food would be nonpoisonous.

After a most delicious seafood luncheon, I rose from the table to thank the boys. The appointed leader or spokesman asked me to wait because there was more to come.

A Thai waiter approached carrying a beautiful celedon plate on which was the piece d'resistance—fourteen fish eyes. At first I didn't think I could manage their gift, but when I looked at those expectant Chinese faces, I decided I'd pretend the eyes were tiny oysters.

To this day, I haven't the foggiest idea how they tasted. I just swallowed each as quickly as I could.

When I'd finished, the lads all stood and applauded, as did almost everyone else in the small restaurant. Apparently not too many Americans tried that delicacy in those days.

* * *

I rummaged in my memory bag today when one of the residents proudly introduced her two granddaughters to me. One was the daughter of her son, the other her daughter's child. I guessed they were about the same age . . . perhaps a year apart. One child was a real little beauty, the other rather nondescript.

I thought of my own childhood when I was about six or seven. An Irish family with two little girls, one a year older than I, the other a year younger, lived near my family home. The two little Irish girls and I were inseparable; we played together by the hour.

My two playmates had black curly hair, large blue eyes, and long, curling lashes.

Whenever anyone passed by the three of us, that person was almost certain to pat one of the little Irish girls on the head and say, "Oh, you pretty little thing." One day, wondering why no one ever patted me on the head saying that, I went to my mother's dressing table, picked up her hand mirror, and surveyed myself from all angles. I saw that my hair wasn't black and it wasn't even curly. Had I known how to describe it, I'd have probably said it was mouse-colored and straight—and no, my eyes were not blue. . . . They were brown and protected by stubby, straight lashes.

I think it was then I first learned I wasn't pretty and that there wasn't much I could do about it.

I don't believe from then on I've ever let my plainness disrupt my life. Of course, there have been times when I wished I were more attractive . . . but then what woman hasn't? I just don't let it bother me.

July 4, 1985

Whenever I returned from any trip abroad, I always felt and said, "Thank God I'm an American." I say it now with even more reverence.

Last evening I watched the Veiled Prophet Parade. Later, I watched the fireworks at the riverfront . . . all on TV, of course.

Although friends asked and were willing to take me to the VP fair, I couldn't see them and/or me—in a wheelchair—facing up to the milling crowd.

⁜   ⁜   ⁜

The aide who assisted me with my whirlpool bath tonight and helped ready me for bed told me that next week she would start work at another nursing home. There surely is some explanation, as this girl has been here four years and seemingly did a good job and was well liked.

Because she was interested in nursing, she has been going to school on her off hours and days. First she studied to become a medical technician, then to become an LPN. Now that she had earned her LPN diploma, she can't understand and is quite hurt that COTG didn't hire her in that capacity.

July 5, 1985

I've learned over the years to look beyond appearances. . . . I try, truly try, to lift my focus beyond what *appears* to me to be the facts.

On two occasions this evening I was reminded to look beyond the obvious. I know that much of our unhappiness is self-inflicted and that before we can be objective in self-appraisal we must first understand and correct those emotions (such as jealousy, hurt pride, anger, or self-pity) that well up in us when things don't go our way.

The nurse aide who is leaving feels rejected, and her pride is terribly hurt.

The silently weeping woman who can't come to terms with her husband's lack of understanding of her physical condition is gradually being consumed by self-pity.

I believe these emotional hurts can only be healed with strength that comes from within. A sympathetic shoulder is but a palliative, placebo, or sugar pill that only soothes a bruised self-esteem. It's only when we become objective that we can put life's happenings into the perspective that gives us the strength to take on the next jolt. And jolts there will be, because that's the secret of living and growing.

July 6, 1985

"Bones of Jade, Soul of Ice, The Flowering Plum in Chinese Art."

Glancing over the invitation to the preview of the above mentioned exhibition at the art museum on July 11, 1985, I know I do want to see this exhibition, perhaps not on the eleventh, but certainly during its stay in St. Louis.

There will be a series of films, lectures by well-known authorities on Chinese art and horticulture, and performances featuring Chinese lion dancers and Chinese puppet theater, to name some of the forthcoming events.

I find this exciting—probably because I'm an admirer of the Chinese, particularly their art and culture.

July 7, 1985

Wasn't it Mark Twain who said he thought God had created man because of his disappointment in monkeys?

I was reminded of that comment when I heard and watched two congressmen debating ways to cut the federal deficit.

Why don't they get on with the job? I believe most Americans know *it must be done and it can't be done without stepping on some toes.* Even though most of us hope it will be the other guy's, we are willing to accept what must be done if it's for the overall good of the country.

July 8, 1985

Emily B—— had grown tired of living in an apartment. About a month or so ago, she bought a little house in Kirkwood. Since then she has had the fun (and hard work) of redoing it.

So that I could see what she has accomplished to date, she invited me to luncheon today. Janet (my private duty aide) transported me, and we spent a delightful afternoon.

Emily has deftly appointed her little home with treasured, but carefully selected, family heirlooms as well as some bibelots and artifacts from her travels. The result is eclectic and charming . . . almost as charming as Emily.

July 10, 1985

Janet T——, my private duty aide, has taken courses in criminal justice at Meramec College and on occasion volunteers her services to the St. Louis County Police Department.

The other day she was commenting about a police incident and I was reminded of two encounters I'd had with criminal justice.

The first took place when I was still able to drive. On the day in question, I was driving north on Twelfth Street when a car pulled out from the curb . . . directly in front of me. I had to slam on my brakes to keep from hitting it. The man driving the car started to put on his hat just as I called out from my lowered window, "Why don't you watch where you're driving?" By the time I'd finished asking that, his police cap was neatly settled on his head. He looked embarrassed, then smilingly said, "Lady, you're right. I should have been more careful. I do apologize!" His reply added to my respect for law enforcement officers.

My other encounter occurred at SBF. I walked into my office one morning to find a strange man looking through my office clothes closet. He was holding one of the heavy hangers I kept there for coats.

In my best "school marm" voice and manner, I demanded that he hand the hanger to me and walk to the door. He did both.

I heard a familiar voice coming from an office down the hallway. Brandishing the coat hanger, I ordered him to head for that office. Why he complied with my every order I'll never know, but he did. I don't think he suspected how scared I was.

I was still waving the heavy wooden hanger around when we arrived at the designated office. The buyer whose voice I heard was using the phone, and I asked if she'd hang up and call for a security guard. I think she sensed I was serious, and she did as I requested.

Within a minute or two a guard bounded down the hallway and I turned over my charge to him . . . all the while hanging onto my coat hanger.

The guard recognized the shoes my intruder was wearing as those belonging to an executive who only the day before had reported to the security office that a very expensive pair of custom-made golf shoes had been taken from his office closet.

A city detective was called, who then took over. He saw the coat hanger, laughed, and asked if I'd come to police headquarters the next day to file and sign certain necessary documents. He then proceeded to give me a lecture I've never forgotten. He told me that if I was ever again in a situation like that I was to do nothing except scream if that was necessary . . . otherwise do nothing! The man might have a knife or gun, et cetera.

Before the detective left my office, he laughingly took my coat hanger, which I was still clutching, and hung it back in the closet. The last I saw, the intruder was in his stocking feet (the guard had taken the shoes), being marched out of my office by the detective.

The next day Morgan went with me to police headquarters, where he and one of the officers were jokingly saying that taxpayers could be saved a great deal of money if police departments purchased coat hangers instead of guns.

I heard later my intruder had only been out of prison three days.

July 11, 1985

There's an undercurrent of discontent seeping into COTG. It surfaces sometimes among the residents . . . at other times among staff members. From my vantage point as a resident, who is cared for by the staff, I really believe a little better secondary supervision would correct almost all of the complaints.

Because complaining is self-feeding and insidious, I hope the director will step in before the situation becomes malignant.

At the moment, the director is busy supervising all the details of the new wing that is under construction and rapidly nearing completion. All of which reminds me of the opening of any new branch . . . whether it's a store or a nursing home wing. There's the planning, construction, decorating, staffing, stocking, and finally the opening of doors for business.

July 12, 1985

Last evening I watched *Casablanca* for the umpteenth time. I tuned into the movie by accident. Thinking there might be a rerun of an old Fiedler concert, this being the one hundredth anniversary of the Boston Pops and not having a TV or radio guide handy, I roamed from channel to channel until I could find something interesting. Not finding a Fiedler or John Williams concert, I settled for *Casablanca.*

It brought back memories of my only trip to Morocco, in the spring of 1972. I was there to buy merchandise for a Mediterranean fair SBF was planning for the fall of 1972. Ron Brummel, display director at SBF at the time, met me in Casablanca. I was to buy the merchandise. Ron was to build the boutiques and create the atmosphere to house the merchandise.

Casablanca when we were there lacked the intrigue and mystery of wartime Casablanca, but 1972 Casablanca and, in fact, Morocco in general held a great fascination for me.

The commissionaire, Ali Bargash, with whom we worked was a son of the former pasha of Rabat. Ali and his attractive wife, Gebida, entertained us in their palace home and introduced us to Ali's older brother and family, with whom we spent an evening. The brother lived in the palace once occupied by the pasha.

The Bargash family motored us to Tangiers, Rabat, Fez, Merrakesh, and other Moroccan towns where Ron and I worked in the souks or medinas. Driving through the Rif one evening at dusk. I found myself humming the music from *Desert Song.* Having purchased Berber jewelry that day, I could hardly avoid thinking of that musical, which I saw for the first time in Chicago when I was a student at Northwestern. The year was 1928, and if I remember correctly, the leading role was sung by Alexander Grey.

In each of the cities we visited, we were usually invited to luncheon or dinner by friends of Ali's. I had my first taste of couscous and a really elaborate Moroccan dinner in Merrakesh.

The souk in Merrakesh was unforgettable, as was a palm-lined avenue there, where I stood looking down on rows of palms to the sands of the Sahara Desert in the near distance and the snowcapped Atlas Mountains in the far distance. I've often wondered how many places are there in the world where from one vantage point one can see lush palm trees, sand dunes, and snowcapped mountains—all at the same time.

July 13, 1985

I recently read a magazine article containing excerpts from an interview with Tom Peters, well-known management consultant and coauthor of that best-selling book *In Search of Excellence.*

So many of his comments regarding lack of perception in industry management seemed to me to be analogous with lack of perception in many facets of health care management.

Some of Peters's cogent remarks were in essence:

1. Everybody talks quality, but it's mostly lip service.
2. The major failure of business is in seeing the employees as part of the problem, instead of as part of the solution.
3. Business is finding out that only half of their problems are external—the rest are internal and self-imposed by management, both top and middle management.
4. Business suffers from an overdose of administrative mentality.

It's too bad managers don't spend some time on the production line. Time so spent is called by business experts "a dose of reality." If exposed to that, most managers would backslide after being promoted to executive positions.

I wonder if nursing home RNs and LPNs wouldn't benefit from a dose of reality or primary care. (Maybe there's a reason hospitals are turning to that.) I have thought for some time that some of our top-notch aides know far more about the care of the residents than the nurses. They're certainly more people-oriented.

July 14, 1985

The Little Red Lighthouse Blues—that's the title of a children's book, which according to a news report was instrumental in saving the little red lighthouse at the foot of New York's George Washington Bridge. Built in 1921, it was to warn Hudson River traffic of the rocky shoreline. When navigational lights were installed on the bridge, there was little use for the lighthouse and plans were made to tear it down. Apparently, the child's story about the little lighthouse saved the day, and the lighthouse will remain as a landmark.

I recall seeing the lighthouse, but mostly I remember the beauty of the George Washington Bridge at night.

To many people, the garland of lights strung the length of the bridge suggested a string of pearls, and it truly looked like that.

I remember crossing the bridge at night to reach Bill Miller's club on the Jersey shore. There, on a moonlit night, the telescoping roof of the club let the stars shine down on the dancers below. Over the years, I spent quite a few pleasant and fun evenings there.

It was at Bill Miller's that Morgan and I first heard Victor Borge. Also, it was there we first heard Eddie Fisher, shortly after Eddie Cantor discovered and sponsored him.

I'm happy the little lighthouse has been saved! If only because it lets me remember so many pleasant evenings.

July 15, 1985

I finally located the correct date and channel, and I watched John Williams and the Boston Pops with guest John Denver last evening. Mickie F—— joined me, as she often does of an evening.

I just finished reading a letter from Renee Robrieux, a long-time friend and very talented Parisienne. She tells me Paris has changed and is changing.

But hasn't and isn't the whole world changed and changing?

- U.S. Navy smuggling and espionage
- Harrods' store-wide half-price sale

- Striking major league baseball players
- Computer milking of cows
- Rock concerts spanning continents to raise money for famine victims
- Sale of Maxim's to Pierre Cardin and his *chain* of Maxim's restaurants
- The increasing number of single-parent households

These are but a few of the situations that are microcosms of a rapidly changing world.

July 16, 1985

I wonder if those who saw CBS's "Night Watch" last night were as amused as I at Alan Simpson's reply to Charlie Rose when Rose asked if he enjoyed being minority whip in the U.S. Senate. Simpson said he thoroughly enjoyed it except when some wag referred to him as "Your Whipship."

July 18, 1985

While searching for a bit of verse my father wrote years ago, I came across the valedictory address I wrote in 1927. I was valedictorian of my graduating class that year at Stivers High School in Dayton, Ohio.

I can remember writing the speech, and I can still remember giving it . . . fifty-eight years ago. I was holding the script in my hands a few minutes ago. It's as I originally wrote it . . . in my handwriting of those long ago days.

I'm going to read it now to see if my thinking and thoughts have progressed or retrogressed in the intervening years.

* * *

Omigod, I've finished reading it (the speech, essay, or whatever it was), and of all the pompous, bloated writing I've ever done, this is the worst. I'm hoping the script I just read was a first draft. I'm inclined to think it might be, as my English teacher's (or somebody's) notations are on the margins . . . a "split infinitive" here . . . a "vague" expression there, et cetera. Surely I must have rewritten this insufferable bit of prose.

As I recall graduation night, I received quite a bit of applause when I finished "speechifying." Maybe the applause was for my parents to keep them from feeling too embarrassed.

The title of my address was "Our Heritage." I still agree with the basic idea I was trying to express, but the way I expressed it (if this was the final draft) . . . well, I was just "too big for my britches," as the expression goes.

July 20, 1985

It was in the seventies . . . some twelve or thirteen years ago.

Because of SBF's interest and active support of the Adopt-a-Pet Program, the Humane Society wanted a picture of Mr. J. A. Baer holding one of the pets. On the day and hour the picture was to be taken, a staff member of the Humane Society, holding a small, wiggling ball of black fluff, and a photographer arrived at Mr. Baer's office. That little ball of charm was called a snoodle (part schnauzer, part poodle). Within minutes, every secretary in the executive offices was oohing and aahing and taking turns holding the small charmer.

The picture was taken, and several of the secretaries thought someone should adopt the little orphan. Mr. Baer had two dogs at the time. Everyone else the girls asked had a pet or pets, lived in an apartment, or had some reason the puppy couldn't be adopted at that time. Knowing I was a bit "dotty" about animals, as one of the secretaries said, the girls kept coming back to me.

Morgan and I had three dogs at the time (a toy poodle, a miniature poodle, and a miniature schnauzer), but once I held that warm, lovable pup in my arms and we exchanged kisses, I succumbed.

We named the new member of our family Samantha, or Sammy for short. She joined the others when we drove to Echo Valley, which we did practically every weekend.

Sammy started to grow up in a hurry. Because she was already larger than our other dogs, she'd curl up on the backseat of the car. The other three stretched out on the front seat between Morgan and me.

Sammy loved Echo Valley Farm. She roamed by the hour. I believe she knew every square foot of the 540 acres.

Bill and Dorothy Counts and their family cared for our cattle and, in general, looked after Echo Valley for us. It wasn't long before Sammy and the Counts children were the best of friends.

Sammy not only grew in personality and charm; she grew in size, too. At first, Morgan and I thought she had to be part *giant* schnauzer and part *standard* poodle (both good-sized dogs). Later, we concluded she was part pony and part mountain goat (she could climb anything) and *all* personality.

Following the loss of Morgan and my stroke, when it became apparent, even to me, that I should go into a nursing home, I still had all four dogs. Bob Cary, who loved animals, took my three little ones. The Counts family took Sammy. I knew all four would be loved and well cared for.

While I've been at COTG, each of the little ones died of old age. They were ten, eleven, and twelve years old.

Two days ago I received a tearful letter from Dorothy Counts telling me Sammy, too, had died in her sleep. Sammy was either twelve or thirteen.

As with the loss of the others, the lump in my throat is very hard to swallow.

July 21, 1985

"Want company?" the friendly resident asked as she opened my door.

"Sure," I answered. "Come in."

Entering, she said, "I'm so lonely I could cry. My son and daughter-in-law are out of town, and I haven't seen any of my old friends for weeks."

It thought, *How fortunate I am that I can be alone and not be lonely. I wonder why?*

Easy, I answered myself. *Because I'm never really alone.*

Aside from my faith, which is always with me, there are the warm and wonderful memories I have and treasure of friends and happenings of bygone years . . . and Morgan, he'll always be a part of me.

How could I forget the challenges we met and overcame? The goals we achieved or the love we felt and shared?

No, I don't think I could ever be really alone.

I wish I could show others that by drawing upon the experiences of their past (some of those experiences are sad, some are downright hilarious, and many are joyful), we could and would smooth today's road and tomorrow's pathway.

How much Morgan and my father would have enjoyed seeing the enactment of the 1905 Dead Horse Hill Climb at Worcester, Massachusetts, last month. I'd have enjoyed it, too! Morgan and Dad, both engineers, always had an interest in cars, classic cars in particular. Perhaps my interest must have come by osmosis.

According to the article I just finished reading in the *Monitor*: "64 horseless carriages of yester-year re-enacted the climb of 1905. One by one, racing against the clock, they throttled up the 1-mile incline, climbing 843.2 feet in height. The winners in 6 classes were: a 1909 Lambert, 1914 Ford, 1912 Buick, 1912 Overland, 1910 Stanley, and 1911 Simplex. The fastest time went to the Stanley . . . 1 minute, 9 seconds . . . the same time as the winning car, also a Stanley, in 1905."

I can remember my dad owning a Stanley Steamer. That could have been in 1912 or 1913. I remember because we (my parents and I) were taking a short trip when a steam coil blew out. The noise shook the countryside, but only I was scared. I know I cried for some time. Apparently blowing a coil in a steam car was not too uncommon in those days.

I don't remember all of the cars, but according to family stories, among the cars my father owned over the years was a 1902 Pope Toledo (forerunner of the Locomobile). I believe it was a steam car, too, and the first west of something or other . . . probably the Mississippi, as my parents were living in Nebraska at the time. According to family stories, also among the many cars he once owned were a white Steamer as well as a Stanley or two.

Because of a car game my dad played with me when I was small, I can still recall names of American-made cars that are uncommon names today.

I wonder how many people remember cars or even names like Abbot-Detroit, Peerless, Graham, Essex, Pierce Arrow, Scrips Booth, Cole, Cord, Stutz Bearcat, Rambler, Dusenberg, Chandler, Mercer, Queen, King, Willys Knight, Jordan Playboy, Flint, Franklin (I know that the Franklin was air-cooled), Cleveland, Maxwell, Durant, Whippet, Moon, Diana, and Dorris. (If I'm not mistaken, the last three originated in St. Louis. The Moon and the Diana were assembled cars and were assembled here, I'm almost certain.)

I believe if I tried, I could recall more names, but back to the article I read referring to the 1905 climb.

The cars driven by steam or internal combustion were given a running start of 200 feet downhill.

After the original races, the participants were given a banquet, then a concert by the Ideal Mandolin Club.

The 1905 climb, first held three years before the first Model T, was considered very dangerous and the ultimate test for cars. Because the "opposition to the speed demons" was growing fierce, the last Dead Horse Hill climb was held in 1911.

P.S. Before I came to COTG, I sold the two remaining classic cars Morgan and I owned. They were a 1927 Star, which he hadn't started to restore, and a 1955 or 1956 (I don't recall which) Thunderbird convertible. The convertible was fun and we loved driving it.

July 25, 1985

Climbing my mountain isn't too difficult when I'm musically motivated, as I was last evening at the St. Louis County Pops.

Richard Hayman conducted the St. Louis Symphony in a memory-stirring evening of Rodgers and Hammerstein. Excerpts from musicals such as *Carousel, State Fair, Oklahoma, South Pacific,* and *The Sound of Music* were played.

I soaked up the music like a sponge and had such a good time recalling and being grateful that my work at SBF required frequent trips to New York, where I had the opportunity to catch most of the Broadway hits between the years 1946 through 1974.

I went to bed last night humming "It's a Grand Night for Singing" and "Climb Every Mountain."

July 25, 1985

Abigail is eighty-seven, saucy and very sure of herself. She was wearing a very short, flouncy nightgown when the aide assisting her to dress asked, "Abby, are you going in for miniskirts now?"

Abby answered, "Of course! I've gone through two husbands, and I see no reason why I shouldn't start looking for a third."

July 26, 1985

I understand any anatomy or physiology textbook will tell me that billions . . . yes, billions of my body cells are renewed every second. Scientists go so far as to say my skin is renewed about every three weeks, my red blood cells are renewed about every four months, and few of my bone cells are more than a year old. In other words, some part of my body is constantly renewing itself. This marvelous renewal, however, does not take place in the brain or central nervous system, and the physical brain should not be confused with the mind. The brain is but a vehicle or tool to be used by the mind.

Knowing this, I want my mind to direct and utilize my brain cells to their fullest capacity. I see no point in letting my mind fill those cells with the debris of resentment, loneliness, fear, or discordant thoughts of any kind. Instead, I'd like to fill them with understanding of others, acceptance and appreciation of all the good that has come my way, and a continuation of my desire to learn.

Midnight—July 26, 1985

I've spent another enjoyable evening at the Pops.

Tonight it was George Gershwin, Jerome Kern, and Irving Berlin music with vocalist Toni Tenile and, of course, the great St. Louis Symphony.

It was a varied program, highlighted here and there with selections such as Dvorak's Slavonic Dance No. 8 and "Malaguena" by Lacuona.

Have a hunch I'll go to sleep humming "I Can't Help Loving That Man of Mine," "Summertime," and "To All the Girls I've Loved Before," the song Julio Iglecius (wonder if I spelled his name correctly?) has made so popular.

July 28, 1985

Today was a full and satisfying day. Emily, Janet, and I had brunch at Schneithorsts', where I met and chatted with Estelle S——, who is still grappling with the hurts of widowhood.

In the afternoon, I watched the Chinese shadow puppet show at the art museum. I was most impressed by the composition and balance of the shadow pictures created or achieved by the puppeteers in each of the miniature dramas they depicted on the screen.

In the evening, Vic and Vickie Harvey stopped by for a brief visit. They're such pleasant people.

July 29, 1985

I don't know how the subject came about, but at luncheon today my tablemates and I discussed ballet. Each one of us, as small girls, had been exposed to ballet, toe, tap, or some form of dancing school training. Each had something to remember about the experience.

My experience was not so much my experience as that of my parents. They, along with other proud parents, were gathered at the evening dance recital to applaud their offspring when each performed.

According to my parents, I danced "beautifully" when I and three other little girls tutued about the stage.

It was only later when the older students were toe dancing that they wanted to disown me or give me to the first passerby.

It seems I was standing slightly in back of a forward wing on the stage, completely oblivious to the fact that I was in full view of the audience. I, dressed as a tiny green elf, was doing my best to imitate the older girls. I was trying to toe dance in my ballet slippers and only succeeded in bobbing up and down like a cork in turbulent water. At first a titter went through the audience. . . . Finally came out and out laughter.

My mother whispered to my father, "Why is everyone laughing? I think the girls are dancing beautifully. Is something wrong?"

My father answered, "Better take another look. That whirling, bobbing comic relief on the right peeking out from the wing is your . . . I mean our kid."

July 30, 1985

I don't understand why some people can't see that the impasse over the federal deficit, the impasse between the president and Congress, is political. . . . It's an impasse between the executive and legislative branches traceable to the *fact* that by law the president cannot run again, whereas the lawmakers must face voters again in '86 and '88.

Looking out for me-me-me seems to be the order of the day. Unfortunately, that order might prevail.

* * *

One of the residents said she had watched an old movie last week. The movie was called *The Amazing Dobermans.*

I immediately thought of the four Dobermans my family owned when I was a girl. The dogs were all pedigreed, with long names stretching from here to there. I remember their call names were Lady, Kay, Donna, and Dixie. They were magnificent creatures: sleek, intelligent, gentle, and fiercely loyal. I've always thought a Doberman given love and kind treatment could be taught to do almost anything. Our four could easily jump or scale a twenty-foot fence, but convincing Timmy of their lovability took a bit longer.

Timmy was the biggest, ugliest, meanest old tomcat I ever saw . . . also the most affectionate.

We first saw Timmy sitting on the lawn one bone-chilling misty-wet fall evening. He just sat there looking over the surroundings. We had no idea from where he came or what he wanted. He just sat. When it started to rain, my father went out to get him, thinking he might be hurt. He wasn't. He just wanted attention. My father named him Timothy Tugmutton, and it wasn't too long before Timmy became a member of the family.

The Dobermans tolerated, even accepted him, but Timmy didn't accept the Dobermans except on his terms. Timmy would wait by a doorway, any doorway through which he thought a Doberman might enter or exit. Timmy just sat looking pleased with himself. Whenever a Doberman came through the doorway, Timmy reached out a long clawed paw. Each Doberman soon carried Timmy's brand . . . a long scratch the length of the dog's nose.

There were never any fights. The Dobermans never lowered their dignity. When Timmy saw he was getting no response, he tired of the game and gave it up. It wasn't too long before the five of them became friends. Timmy would often curl up alongside any one of the Dobermans and go to sleep.

July 31, 1985

Last night I was the classic example of the inmate trying to run the asylum. It was two o'clock in the morning, and for the third time (once on the morning shift, again on the evening shift, and then on the night shift) the hall aide brought a new girl or trainee into my room to observe or "orientate," as all the aides say. Whether the word is *orient* (orient—to adjust to or condition to a situation, as Webster says) or *orientate* is irrelevant. What is relevant is that the new trainee (as did the other two new girls) just stood like a zombie gazing around the room while the aide went about her business of transferring me. I thought it was about time someone did a little teaching.

So I took it upon myself to explain why I had to be lifted a certain way . . . that I was paralyzed on the left side. I explained about the foot surgery I'd had and why I had to sleep with a cast on my leg and a splint on my hand at night, et cetera.

All I did was upset everyone! The hall aide later wanted to know if I was annoyed with her for not explaining. I told her no, but I thought it time someone did a little showing and telling as each trainee was introduced to a resident.

Even the charge nurse came to my room later to find out what was wrong. I told her the same thing I told the aide . . . that a little explanation along with "hoisting" me would do much to orient the new girl—at least as far as I was concerned. And it seems I upset the trainee, too, telling her that *if* my paralyzed arm was pulled it might slip out of its socket (as has happened) because of weakened muscles. I jokingly said that if she did that when learning to transfer me, I wouldn't let her come back into the room. That must have scared her or offended her, as the aide told me later the trainee was upset and didn't think she wanted to be an aide.

From now on, I'll be the inmate who leaves the training to the nurses and aides, who in my opinion do a far from adequate job of it. But then who asks for my opinion?

In retrospect . . . maybe I didn't do the wrong thing in trying to do a bit of teaching. The trainee on the day shift later came back to thank me for my efforts. The aide on the evening shift immediately picked up on the explanations when she heard what I was attempting to do.

It was only on the night shift that I struck out!

August 1, 1985

I'm ashamed to say I've never once wondered about the expression "once in a blue moon." If I ever thought about it at all, I probably dismissed the idea of a "blue moon" being as factual as the idea of the moon being made of "green cheese."

It wasn't until yesterday, July 31, that I learned the blue moon expression came from the fact that only once in three years does a full moon appear twice in any one month. . . . Then the moon is called blue . . . even though it's as shiny bright as a newly minted dollar.

On July 2 and July 31, 1985, a full moon appeared. Not until 1988 will a full moon appear twice in one month. Then it will be during the month of May 1988.

Now I'm beginning to wonder about the expression "the moon is made of green cheese." I have a haunting suspicion it might come from some fairy tale or bit of folklore. Guess I'll do some sleuthing.

Well, I sleuthed and found that Thomas Moore used the expression back in the 1400s. Whether it was used before that I didn't learn. I did find out, however, that following Moore, Thomas Heywood, also an Englishman, in his collection of sayings and proverbs referred to the expression, but very carefully explained the moon really wasn't green, that it was in reality *new*. He further explained that the expression was borrowed from the cheesemakers, who referred to green cheeses, which often are crescent-shaped, as *new* and not aged.

Now wouldn't common sense have explained that bit of trivia to me? It didn't, but the public library did. I have an idea the gracious lady who helped me by phone with my sleuthing probably thought I should hang up and rearrange the rocks in my head.

August 3, 1985

For almost seven years I've been working on a mosaic . . . a mosaic I'm carefully putting together with broken pieces and fragments of a life I once knew. My mosaic is emerging, I hope, as a pleasing picture worthy of my heritage, Morgan, and those friends who never once lost confidence in my ability to cope and adjust to a strange me and a sometimes tearful existence in a nursing home.

The broken pieces I've picked up to polish and include in this picture of my thinking and life today are culled from memorable moments from the past, encouraging words from friends, bits of wisdom from the many books I've read, yes, and unforgettable scenes from my travels such as the awe and thrill I experienced when I saw (and felt I could almost touch) Mount Everest from the cabin of a Royal Nepal plane . . . or the languid twilights viewed from a houseboat on Kashmir's Dall Lake . . . or the uncomfortable hardness of a waiting room bench in the Tokyo airport when, due to a delay in Kathmandu, I missed all of my flight connections and couldn't get a room in Tokyo at three o'clock in the morning, but I used my flight bag as a pillow, my coat as a blanket and slept quite well. I think I was too tired to know whether I slept or not.

There's a little bit of everything in my mosaic. . . . It's a montage of happiness and sadness, laughter and tears, excitement and boredom, of friends old and new, of regret and anticipation, and it's all held together with a cement made of upbeat thoughts and of love freely given and received.

During the making of this mosaic, a kind of personal philosophy has evolved.

Strange that a nursing home has become my Walden's Pond.

August 5, 1985

While listening to Joan Baez singing with the Boston Pops last evening, I kept thinking, *American fado?* I'm sure I'm not the first person to notice the similarity between American folk or narrative songs and Portuguese fado; however, that similarity struck me more forceably last night than it ever had before. Whether it was the poignant quality of Baez's voice or the plaintive words of the ballads I don't know. . . .

Some country western has an element of the same pathos, I suppose, but it has never impressed me as being similar to fado. American fado?

August 6, 1985

All because I watched National Geographic's salute to Sir Edmund Hillary last evening I've been thinking all day of Nepal, that tiny kingdom high in the towering Himalayas, Kathmandu its capital, and the kind, likable Nepalese people.

I made two trips to Nepal in the early seventies, and I can visualize to this day Kathmandu, like fabled Xanadu nestling in a fertile valley of the high Himalayas. At first the city seemed to me like something out of dreams. The soft muted colors of the ancient shrines, the pagoda-type temples, the medieval buildings with their hand-carved doors and window frames contrasted with the gaily colored animal carvings and the Tanric erotic art on the supporting struts of the temples. Every piece of available wood seemed to be carved and colored.

I remember early one morning watching from my hotel window the sun seeping through and beginning to clear the mist that hung like a fleecy cloud over the valley. It wasn't long before the gilded

Toran and "The Eyes of Badnath," high on a hill overlooking Kathmandu, came into view. The centuries-old buildings slowly took shape, and the quiet dawn was soon shattered by the cacophony of daylight sound. I recall the crowing of roosters and the voices of workmen calling to one another . . . the sign a new day was beginning.

After I retired from SBF, I planned to revisit Nepal. As I never made it, I'm doing it now in memory. I'm being helped along in that by looking at a wedding invitation Morgan and I received from N. G. Joshi, inviting us to attend a double wedding ceremony. A son and daughter were to be married on March 5, 1976. If Morgan hadn't been ill at the time of the double wedding and if it wasn't to take place on the other side of the world, I'm pretty sure Morgan and I would have attended—or made an attempt to do so.

Now I'm remembering houses of rust-colored brick closed in by roads of brick tile set in chevron pattern where only people, trishaws, hand-pushed carts, and an occasional cow traveled. I can almost smell the sweet, aromatic incense that hung heavy in the air over the old part of town and see people bargaining, praying, talking, or just sitting. The men dressed in labeda surwals (the high-collared shirts worn outside their trousers) with tails flapping. All wore a Western-style jacket over the shirt. The women wore sarong-type skirts or saris and carried or watched their bare-bottomed tots playing in the street. All wore golden earrings.

And how can I forget the yak and yeti or the legendary Boris, the Russian who turned a palace into a hotel, the Sherpas, Genesh (the elephant god)—there's so much to recall and I'm so tired of remembering. So enough for now.

August 7, 1985

Last evening I spent another enjoyable two hours at the County Pops. The audience gave Roger Williams three standing ovations. Richard Hayman and Williams apparently struck the right informal note, as I've never seen the symphony or a performer at the Pops received with more enthusiasm . . . loud enthusiasm.

Of course, Williams played "Autumn Leaves" and "September Song." The Chopin selections he chose were, I thought, beautifully executed.

August 9, 1985

I'm enough of a realist to know that in all likelihood it will be necessary for me to spend the rest of my life in and out of a wheelchair, living in a nursing home or in an apartment of my own with nursing care.

The new COTG annex is rapidly taking form and will be ready for occupancy within the next two or three months. That means I must soon decide whether I want to stay where I am, in my spacious room, move into the new annex where the rooms I understand are smaller, or rent an apartment and hire my own nursing help.

I like the room I have but am not too happy with the character of the hall on which it's located.

Whatever I decide, I want it to be my last move. For that reason, there must be a consensus between my head, my heart, and my wallet. *I must think this through carefully.* Like everyone else, I don't know whether my life tenure will be for another two weeks, two months, two years, or twenty years.

I only know that if I can avoid it, I do not want or intend to become a physical or financial burden to anyone.

That's why I keep telling myself that my mind, my heart, and my wallet must all be in agreement regarding my future.

August 10, 1985

I have watched more television since coming to COTG than I ever watched in all the years before. I once thought most television programs were a waste of time. I found radio more interesting because I could keep informed and still move about. I couldn't understand sitting in one spot with my eyes glued to the boob tube, as it was often called then.

Today, because of my lack of mobility and the restricted life I live, I've found that by carefully choosing my programs I can keep my horizons broadened, my various interests heightened . . . and often I'm able to touch base with my past.

I watched the TV coverage of the St. Louis Centre opening.

It appeared impressive and I'm glad it was a success. . . . However, I'm looking forward to the opening of the new Union Station mall with much more interest. Had a Stix, Baer and Fuller store anchored one side of the Centre (rather than Dillards) I'm certain I'd be more enthusiastic about the Centre. You can't work for and love a company as I did for thirty-three years without feeling a tug at your heart when you finally realize the company is no more.

I knew SBF when it was a family-owned, quality fashion store. It was a people-oriented organization, loved by its employees. Then it was a profitable operation, which was the reason Associated Dry Goods (ADG) bought it when a dissident member or two of the family forced its sale.

Not knowing or rather not comprehending that St. Louis is a charming, cultured small town, ADG sent sophisticated New Yorkers here to manage the SBF stores. A succession of presidents from the East did nothing but muff the operation, to the point where it was losing money and ADG sold that wonderful old store to Dillards.

Dillards I'm sure is a good organization. It too is family-owned, but by a computer-oriented family, in my opinion. (I'll admit I'm prejudiced.)

I'm happy it was my privilege to work in retailing when the customer was right, if not always, at least most of the time.

Old Stix, Baer and Fuller cared about people, customers, employees, resources, and St. Louis.

I have a notion there are thousands of St. Louisans who feel as I do about the demise of SBF.

August 11, 1985

Today I visited a lovely, beautifully appointed and equipped retirement complex. Were I ambulatory, I'd be very tempted to move there at once. But I'm not and while I have no intention of negatively programming my physical situation, I'm hesitant to move so quickly. My ambivalence is due to:

1. My present need for more nursing care (much as I want to be more self-reliant). Physically, I know I'm not ready as yet to be so much on my own.
2. I want to see what the new COTG annex has to offer.
3. I want to check the nursing home care and facilities of the retirement complex I visited.
4. I want to compare carefully the nursing home facilities of COTG with the other.
5. Because of the care I've received at Clayton-on-the-Green for over six years, I can't in all conscience make any final

decision without first discussing with Mrs. Bono, COTG director, all my reasons for even considering a move.

I ended this soul-searching day by sorting out my thoughts and emotions by listening to the Boston Pops. The duo pianists, the talented French girls Kathe and Marinelle DeBeque, were guest artists. Their rendition of Gershwin's *Rhapsody in Blue* helped me do the sorting.

August 12, 1985

COTG's river cruise today on the *President* brought back memories of Morgan's and my boating days on the Ol' Mississippi. No two people had more relaxation, enjoyment, and just plain fun than we did . . . moonlit nights on the river . . . daylight lounging on a sandbar barbecuing, often with friends . . . cruises up the river to Chicago and Lake Michigan . . . downriver to Kentucky Lake and other resort ports of call. Yesterday's brief but pleasant cruise brought it all back, happily. It was a long day in a wheelchair, but tired as I was when we docked, I enjoyed every minute of it, and when I was tucked in for the night, I couldn't help thinking how I've been blessed all my life.

August 14, 1985

With a world in turmoil it was comforting to pick up a newspaper and read about a Swiss agronomist who believes in life and growth rather than destruction and devastation. Rene Haller has spent twenty-five years in East Africa. According to Haller, no terrain is so devastated that something can't be done about it. To prove his theories that a viable concern can operate and still contribute to environmental management, Haller established an experimental farm on the exhausted land of the Bamburi Portland Cement Company, which had laid waste vast tracts of bushland as it extracted millions of tons of limestone along Kenya's beautiful Indian Ocean coast.

From acres of hard splintered coral and silica refuse he produced seventy acres of reforestation with one-hundred-foot-high trees, teeming fish ponds, and lush meadows.

How he accomplished it is a fascinating story and one everyone who is interested in nature and the environment might want to investigate.

No wonder Rene Haller is now an independent adviser to the United Nations Food and Agriculture Organization. Surely there has been a book or two written about him. I plan to call the public library and inquire.

August 15, 1985

Elvira and Belle are tablemates. Both are in their eighties and on special diets. Elvira, who is inclined to be bossy, *accepts* her salt-free diet, but complainingly. Belle, who is overweight and a bit rebellious, *objects* to her calorie-counted diet complainingly. I sit near them and can't help but overhear most of their mealtime conversations.

Yesterday Belle was fussing about her dish of Jell-O while having to watch others enjoy their chocolate eclairs.

Elvira, annoyed, said, "Drink your coffee while it's hot and move your glass of water or you'll push all your utilities on the floor."

Belle glaringly answered, "If you mean my utensils, my glass of water isn't near them."

Elvira countered with, "Utensils are pots and pans and are in your kitchen, not here."

With that I excused myself from the table, and I don't know who won that verbal bout.

August 16, 1985

I was asked today by one of my friends how I *really* liked living in a nursing home. I thought for a moment and replied, "If I borrowed the words 'between tears and laughter,' the title of one of Lin Yutang's books, I believe that best describes my feelings about institutional living."

But, upon further thought, isn't that the normal state of the universe and of the human mind and body? Isn't there always that swing between extremes? Isn't there always a rhythmic action and reaction?

The day follows night, the tide ebbs and flows, the moon waxes and wanes, and the seasons follow in an orderly fashion. We humans, in fact, all living organisms, inhale and exhale; hearts beat and pause; we are in turn active and passive.

My reaction to life depends on how I accept the vicissitudes of daily living. Do I accept? Do I reject? How *I* adjust determines the quality of my life. And as I've always admired quality (using quality in the real sense of the word), I can truthfully say that nursing home living hasn't deterred my enjoyment of life.

August 18, 1985

August 1985—forty years this month World War II finally ended with the surrender of Japan. With all the media coverage, both retrospective and contemplative, and with my thinking about *Between Tears and Laughter,* I was reminded how impressed I was with that book, which was published not too long after the war ended, so I've been rereading it.

How prophetic Lin Yutang was and how perceptive his comments. Following are some of those cogent comments:

> We cannot escape history.
> The invisible forces of history are breaking up the international structure of our world. Politically we ignore them.
> We are sowing what we do not mean to reap.
> Even the smallest act has its consequences.
> We cannot escape from the chain of accusation.
> There are a rhythm and a pattern of things in human history if only we could detect them.
> There are more historical analogies than we can stomach.
> The great thing about the teaching of history is that we must teach history but must not let history teach us.

In Lin Yutang's section on the suicide of Greece, he says: "One could wish that Athenian and modern parallels were less exact."

I could go on, but this is a book one should read and reread for oneself. I hope politicians around the world will become acquainted with it or the message Lin Yutang is trying to get across. They, the politicians, might even take a peek into Barbara Tuchman's *March of Folly.*

August 19, 1985

I watched and listened to a debate on the ethics of euthanasia last night. The arguments stirred up feelings and a conviction of my own. Being mentally alert, or at least I've been told so, I hope the wishes I express now will be respected if I ever become a burden, physically or financially or heart-wise, to anyone.

1. I do not wish to be kept alive by means of any kind of life support system.
2. If I should be beyond knowing or become unable to speak for myself or become a nuisance or care to anyone, I sincerely hope a doctor, the hospital, or someone will "pull the plug" or give my life termination an assist. Only my body, which I consider but a shell, will be destroyed.

I've said many times I have no fear or apprehension about death. What I do fear is that I won't be permitted to die with dignity.

August 20, 1985
"What a difference a thought makes."

I wish I had said that, because I know so well the power and energy of thoughts. A thought can be a pulsating, vibrant bit of loving energy that reaches out to others or it can be a selfish, moody cry in the night that closes doors.

I have learned that my thoughts determine my attitude and that my attitude determines how I feel. Therefore, how I feel is usually up to me!

At the moment, I'm feeling a bit sad. My likable, competent private duty aide, Janet, is in the throes of a stressful divorce and is moving away. As of the first of September, she'll be leaving me. While I'm unhappy at the thought of losing her, I'm more unhappy about what the divorce is doing to her. She has become moody and no little sorry for herself. I had hoped she and her husband could and would work out their differences. Apparently not. As I believe each person has the right to live his own life, all I can say to her is, "I'm sorry and I'll truly miss you."

August 23, 1985
A sense of humor . . . what a wonderful, desirable attribute to have. I think one of the many reasons I admire Ronald Reagan as I do is due to the fact that no matter what is thrown at him, he almost always fields it well and smilingly. I can think of several occasions when I thought his spontaneous answers to hurtful statements or questions were inspired.

There was the time during the 1984 presidential organization campaign when the Democrats' nominee for vice president, Geraldine Ferraro, in one of her speeches accused Reagan of not being a Christian. Later when a reporter asked the president how he responded to that, Reagan replied, "Why, I just turn the other cheek."

On another occasion, when Prime Minister Nakasone of Japan remarked at a state dinner in Washington that it was difficult to lose an entire city—he was referring to Hiroshima. I understand that Mr. Reagan suggested that he take a look at Detroit.

Last evening at a fund raising dinner in California, Mr. Reagan's first public appearance out of the White House since his operation, the president commented about all the letters he has received during his convalescence. He laughingly read one he particularly liked. It said in essence, "Mr. President, I'm told you had two feet removed from your inner workings. Tell me, sir, how did those two feet get in there in the first place?"

I keep thinking, *How can you keep the likes of a president or the American people, in general, down when no matter what happens, they get up, dust themselves off, laugh a bit (usually at themselves), and keep on keeping on?*

That spirit is hard to beat!

If a mile is 5,280 feet, then I'm walking (mechanically, of course, with my steel brace and cane) over one mile and a quarter each month. I walk approximately 240 feet daily up and down my hallway. That is 1,640 feet weekly or 6,720 feet every four weeks. One and a quarter miles is only sixty-six hundred feet.

I hope my friends won't mind if I feel a mite smug and pleased with myself.

*　*　*

I have been sniffling, snuffling, wheezing, and tenderly mopping my runny nose all morning. The rain, the allergy count, and my sinuses are anything but compatible. My runny eyes and nose remind me of a story about a little girl on her first day of school.

The teacher asked all the youngsters to be seated, explaining that she'd come to each one, get his or her name, and later arrange the permanent seating.

Turning to the first little girl, she said, "Now, dear, what is your name?"

110

The child replied, "Snotty."

The teacher, a bit startled, said, "No, dear, that can't be. Now tell me your real name."

The youngster kept insisting that her name was Snotty. Finally, the exasperated teacher told her that she would have to go home to get a note from her parents stating her name.

The little girl was indignant. She stomped to the door, and as she opened it, a small boy skidded through. The little girl called to him, "You might as well go home, Shitty. She won't believe you either."

I know, I know, the story isn't very delicate, and it may not even be funny, but my soggy head made me think of it.

August 25, 1985

Whether my hurts are physical or emotional, I seldom let them surface. . . . However, at the moment I'm not doing a very good job of hiding those hurts . . . from others, yes, but not from myself. I know my feelings are hurt because of the inconsideration of another. That, coupled with the discomfort of sinusitis, has turned this day into a bummer of a day.

If I'm as good as I think I am about controlling the direction of my attitudes, then I should be able to turn this zero day into something approaching a ten. . . .

Later

I didn't quite make it to ten . . .

August 26, 1985

But I did go to sleep laughing last night.

When I moved into COTG, I brought with me enough books to fill two large bookcases in my room. They were all books I wanted to reread.

On my way to bed last night, I picked out Dr. Joseph Peck's *Life with Women and How to Survive It.*

I reread and chuckled until midnight.

Dr. Peck's book is hilarious, uninhibited, witty, and a must for anyone, man or woman, who thinks he or she knows women.

When I finish *Life with Women,* I intend to re-read Dr. Peck's *All About Men.* It's equally delightful, entertaining, and refreshing.

August 28, 1985

More about Dr. Peck's book, *Life with Women.*

Just as I felt many of Lin Yutang's statements were perceptive, I believe the following quotes from Dr. Peck are worth repeating:

There are a lot of similarities between the battle of the sexes and the cold war we have been enjoying with the Russians. Russia has adopted the female technique for keeping her adversary off balance down to the last comma, and Uncle Sam has shown the perfect picture of the bewildered male in his reactions.

The courtship went on during the last World War. Uncle Sam showered gifts upon this new-found partner, and received kind and gentle words of love from Russia, but she showed no disposition to bestow any gifts of love in return. The beautiful romance was pictured at Yalta by Russia, and our old uncle lapped it up, despite the warnings of that elder brother, England. At Potsdam, the suitor fell for the age-old trick of deeding over half of his property to his lady love before he got her name on the dotted line. Since that time, it's been the usual course of married love, the wife blowing hot and cold by turns, and the husband totally confused by her changes of mood. Sometimes she is in the "how-dare-you" stage, a woman wronged. "How could you treat me so, you brute!" But when she wants to work the mixed up husband for a new mink coat, along will come the forgiving smile and tears and once more he will awake in the morning nicely situated in the doghouse with his pockets picked again.

The similarity between our government's actions and that of its own male citizens goes even further. There was a time when this country was gloriously masculine, tending to its own business and insisting that others do the same. But the depression of the thirties changed its character to such an extent that even our creator must have developed grave doubts of its sanity.

The American male cast off his natural gift of being the architect of his own fortune, and with a mighty sigh of relief, placed his dependence for his old age on the mighty shoulders of F.D.R. and got the Social Security Act. A man with a spark of initiative left in his soul was cast as an undesirable character and not allowed to work to support his family unless he would accept serfdom. As this is reflected in the individual citizen, his natural masculine nature is so tamed that his only desire is to get into a labor union that will do his thinking for him, or a company which supervises his every action, even the choice of his wife, all so that he may enjoy his social security, pension, sick insurance, and all the other gimmicks classed under the broad skirts of security.

Every time modern man accepts some government handout, he loses just so much of his masculine individuality. Thirty long years of father image with the brief interlude when Harry tried unsuccessfully to instill some old stubborn mulishness into us has just about plucked all the tail feathers from the American eagle and now the damn thing has begun to cluck!

August 29, 1985

Of course Dr. Peck exaggerates, but in my opinion there's an element of truth in all that he says.

I once thought I was an independent thinker politically. But I'm not! At least not now. Analyzing my reaction to political issues over the years, I find I cozy up to the philosophy of the Republican party.

I so firmly believe it isn't what government can do for the American people but what the American people can do for themselves. I believe that's the credo that built and made this country great! I also believe our people today are smart enough and have enough initiative to overcome our industrial and labor problems and be able to compete with any other peoples of the world. For that reason, I believe in free trade and less government interference. I do not favor protectionism.

August 31, 1985

It's time I climbed down from my soapbox. Besides, who cares what an oldster living in a nursing home thinks about free trade, free enterprise, tax reform, federal deficit, and other oddments? . . . Better I "should" read a book, listen to some music, take a labored walk down the hallway . . . anything to keep from boring others with my opinions. Fortunately, I write down most of those opinions and don't "spout off" verbally too often.

Because I don't want to retrogress therapy-wise, I should intensify my efforts in finding a good private duty aide. Today is Janet's last day. She has helped more with follow-up therapy than any aide I ever had.

September 1, 1985

I learned yesterday while listening to a discussion on technological development that "any 17-year-old today has seen more advances in technology in his short lifetime than have taken place in all the years before . . . and that there's more to come."

Whenever I hear or read something like that, it's the only time I wish I had my life ahead of me. I think I'd have a marvelous time. Not that I regret the past. My past has given me the stamina and courage to face up to and accept my life today. Not that there aren't days when I want to lay back my ears and bray. There are! Yes, and get on my soapbox. For example, I'd like to spank the young people today who won't work at making marriage a success. It was the hardest job I ever had and by far the most rewarding!

Whenever I rummage in my files, I come up with something I knew should be there, something I have felt but haven't seen in years. Today it was a rejection slip for a story I wrote and sent to *Redbook* Magazine. I don't recall the year, and I don't know if that magazine is even in existence today. Along with the story were bits of free verse I wrote at different times to Morgan during our marriage. Following are two of those bits of my versifying:

> I talk to you of many things
> You never hear me say
> And yet you understand.
> It must be we have built
> A silence of familiarity
> On which our thoughts may cross
> On softly stepping feet.
> There is no space so wide
> We cannot leap across
> And walk together on that pathway
> Of our mind's projection.
> Words may stimulate a marriage
> But it lives and grows strong
> In silence that does not require a voice.
> Written 11/26/38

There are things that I shall keep now that you are gone:
Things I have received from knowing you.
Things you could not lose by giving them away;
The brilliance of a smile not overused,
A charming sense of humor that does not shout
And stand upon a chair and wave its arms.
The dignity of disciplined emotions
And the gracefulness of a mind that seldom stumbles.
A certainty that doesn't wander into pathways,

But walks along the road against the wind
With a stride that could not fail to reach the top
Where cool sunshine turns the grass from green to gold.
                    Written 11/26/78

September 2, 1985

I recently received an informative letter regarding elderly parents from the Research Institute of America. I'm going to forward it to Mrs. Bono. She may be interested in sharing the information with families who have parents in or about to enter a nursing home. I don't have that responsibility but others do. According to RIA, this is a critical family problem that is a "ticking time bomb" for millions of Americans.

There is a book available at $3.95 called *Caring for Dependent Parents.* According to the advertising blurb, the book explores in depth the three kinds of challenges that are involved when you have dependent parents, namely:

1. The financial and legal challenges.
2. The challenges of providing good care.
3. And very important, the psychological challenges not only in handling the stress of the changes made in the parents' life-style, but how to deal with your own stress and guilt.

I'm certainly not on anyone's payroll to push this book, but it sounds to me as though it contains a great deal of helpful information.

I'm going to give the following address to several people I know in the event they are interested:

The Research Institute of America, Inc.
Department 94103
Mount Kisco, NY 10549

I see so much heartache, both family-wise and resident-wise, in a nursing home, I thought perhaps a book like this might help.

Of course, I could be wrong. If so, it won't be the first time.

September 3, 1985

I've been looking at two figurines I purchased in Alghero, that loveliest of Sardinian towns. I made a trip to Sardinia in the early seventies to buy handcrafted items for SBF.

Sardinia is an island with a landscape wrinkled with Basalt Mountains and a seacoast with miles of sugar-white-sand beaches. My trip to Sardinia remains in my memory as another delightful experience.

Many things stand out. . . . The charming hotel where I stopped was built on a rocky projection overlooking the sea. It was a building supposedly once frequented by European royalty. It could have been, as many of the furnishings were quite elegant.

The Sardinian people intrigued me, particularly those I saw on my only trip to the inland town of Nuoro. En route there, I saw several barefooted women, each balancing a water jug on her head, and men with black-scarfed headdresses who smoked and talked in groups in the various villages.

I suppose all this is changed today. The colorful regional costumes were still being worn in most areas. The much publicized banditti were scarce and confined themselves to hilltop vendettas.

En route to one of the villages not too far from Alghero, the commissionaire with whom I was working and I stopped at a wayside inn for a cool drink and a bite to eat. The owner turned out to be the sister of a bandit who had been caught the day before. She, like her brother, was a very independent Sard and seemed quite pleased with the publicity her brother had received.

In that village, I bought a beautiful hand-carved briar pipe for Morgan. Unfortunately, it and a handsome meerschaum from Turkey were never seen after I broke up my home. However, I still have the remains of a box of cork stationery from Sardinia. I had oak cork shaved into razor thin sheets and envelopes and had them beautifully boxed as an exclusive item for SBF. While I don't have the meerschaum pipe Morgan loved and smoked until it was a soft golden brown in color, I still have a hand-hammered copper Byzantine trayed container (once used for carrying food to men working in the fields) that is over six hundred years old.

Many material things have been lost or taken, but my memories of an unusual island with its *nuraghi* (those beehive-shaped watchtowers dating back to 3000 B.C.) still remain.

September 4, 1985

I've learned to overlook most disappointments. However, I don't believe I should overlook the one concerning my therapy. I've had to start over so many times I know I'd be foolish not to make every effort to continue my therapy at the pace I have been going.

For many months (even years) the COTG physical therapist (sometimes a man, sometimes a woman) has worked with me five days a week. I have progressed to the point where the current therapist felt her treatments could be cut back to two times a week. Then Janet's follow-up with me was so good the therapist felt I only needed her one session a week.

With Janet gone and I not yet having an aide who can walk me daily, I asked the therapist if she would be able to increase my treatments to three times a week. She wasn't certain because of her full schedule, but was going to check with the nursing director and my doctor to see what could be worked out. In the event I can't locate an aide quickly, I may find it necessary to have a private therapist. At this point, I'm willing to do whatever is necessary.

September 5, 1985

Next week I start with the physical therapist on a schedule of three times a week until I can locate an aide.

September 6, 1985

The other day I watched a documentary on the all-American raccoon, that delightful little animal that is part thief, part pest, and completely captivating. I was remind of Bandit—the raccoon that came to dinner at Echo Valley . . . and stayed and stayed. Bandy, as we affectionately called him, frequently ensconced himself in the crotch of a large tulip tree outside our screened-in patio. Always in the mornings and often during the day, we exchanged greetings, we calling him by name, he waving his handlike paws in return.

We often saw him fishing in the shallows of a nearby gurgling creek. We soon learned that he liked minnows and crayfish or craw-dads as the countryfolk call them.

Bandy stayed with us all one summer. It was late fall before he left to join his kind. We missed him as we did any and every creature, domestic or wild, that spent time with us. I often thought they some-how sensed that Morgan and I both had love and great respect for all animals.

*   *   *

117

Then there was Lulu, the buffalo Morgan bought from Grant's Farm. Lulu only weighed eight hundred pounds when she came to Echo Valley, but like Sammy, she grew and grew! Eventually she mated with our pedigreed bull Hereford, and before we knew it, we had cattelos—who, not having read the book about hybrids, continued to breed, until we had a couple of generations of like or line producing cattelos.

Lulu became as tame as anything wild and weighing fifteen hundred pounds could be. She was that weight when she was shot by some unknown trigger-happy hunter.

When Morgan found her body, that was the only time I ever saw him really angry.

September 9, 1985

Following my therapy walk this morning and while catching my second breath, I leafed through Rebecca McCann's *Cheerful Cherub,* that whimsical, humorous "hits you where you live" book of sayings and drawings of an unforgettable cherub.

Sometimes the cherub is flip, sometimes sarcastic, but always truthfully pointing out our human frailties.

Of the thousand and one cherubic verses, the following are a few of my favorites:

Empty Head

I'm trying to empty my mind
Of every thought foolish and small—
I wonder if then I shall find
There's nothing left at all.

Evolution

To complain because life isn't perfect
Seems captious and petty of soul—
When you think the world started with chaos
It did pretty well on the whole.

Exaggeration

I cut my finger with a knife.
I neither wept nor moaned nor swooned,
In fact the courage that I showed
Was worthy of a larger wound.

Explosion

When everything goes dead wrong
And fate presses down on my load,
Am I noble and brave?
No, I break things and rave—
It's such a relief to explode.

Faces

We'd find each face was beautiful,
However plain it seems.
If, looking past the dull outside.
We saw the wistful dreams.

Eyes

One thing when sorrow comes to me
Has helped my spirit rise—
The quiet courage that I see
In other people's eyes.

Fretting

I ought to have more faith in life,
Not fret because I'm far from strong,
But do the day's work as I can,
And life will carry me along.

Friendship

Whenever I am plunged in woe
My true friends rally round,
So trouble is a friendship test
If nothing else I've found.

Gain

They say that youth's the carefree time
But I have learned with age this truth:
It's just by growing old we gain
The wisdom to enjoy our youth.

Giving

It's not by hoarding wealth or love
That man grows rich, I see—
The more I freely give to life
The more life gives to me.

Camouflage

Anger at another's fault
I cannot honestly condone.
It's nearly always just a way
To turn attention from my own.

Christmas Boxes

How lovely Christmas boxes look
All holly-trimmed and ribbon-tied
It's often quite a shock to see
The funny things that are inside.

Inner Life

Nothing that happens can hurt me
Whether I lose or win—
Though life may be changed on the surface
I do my main living within.

Climbing

To climb a mountain to the sky
Is easier for me
Than struggling from the way I am
To how I want to be.

Clouds

Each kind heart is like a sun
That shines upon the passing crowd—
How sad I feel on selfish days
When I have lived behind a cloud.

Companions

I wish my dog could talk to me
With thoughts his eyes are big and dark
How sociable our days would be
If he could speak or I could bark!

Complaints

When I complain it often means
No matter how I rage and whine,
I'm really blaming all the world
For faults I will not face as mine.

Compliments

No compliment that I receive
Seems undeserved to me—
I see myself, not as I am
But as I want to be.

Conscience

Sometimes at night my conscience wakes
With pangs it seems that naught can lull
If I could always feel like this
How good I'd be, and oh, how dull!

Consequences

It's foolish to regret mistakes
For everybody makes them
The consequences matter not
As much as how one takes them.

Cowardice

Although I'm brave enough I'm sure
To meet life's gravest situations
I lack the courage to refuse
My dull friends' dinner invitations.

Decisions

Whenever a problem comes up in my life
I decide it and promptly forget it—
It isn't so much the decision that counts
As the willpower not to regret it.

Determination

Although my way seems hard
I'll waste no strength in crying—
For no one ever failed
Unless he gave up trying.

Diaries

The humble part I play in life
Does not much help my self-esteem
But in the diary I keep
You'd be surprised how grand I seem.

Disagreement

When a thoughtful eye I cast
O'er my long disastrous past
I must admit I seldom see
My principles and acts agree.

September 10, 1985

Rereading Rebecca McCann's verses made me think what a special Christmas gift this old book would make for some of my friends.

Knowing the book was out of print but knowing too there were companies that specialized in carrying out-of-print books, I started calling book departments and bookstores to find one that would conduct the search for me. Naturally, I expected to pay both for the books and the service.

To my surprise, none of the shops I called offer that service today. One shop was kind enough, however, to give me the name and address of a company that I could write. another was gracious enough to give me the name of a local shop that for a small fee might help me. I'm determined enough to buy these books if they're available that I'm mailing my request and check to the small shop. Maybe larger shops don't need that kind of business today.

When I merchandised the book department at SBF (that was some ten or twelve years ago), special orders and requests like this added many extra dollars to the department's volume. Sometimes it was a nuisance, but that was retailing as I knew it. Times have certainly changed!

September 12, 1985

Another young couple I know have separated. That makes me wonder if there aren't times when the things we don't say are more hurtful and do more harm than our spoken words. I'm thinking of a forgotten "Thank you" to someone who is working hard to please you or the silent *I love you* to someone who feels neglected.

Angry words if coming from someone who is ill, hurting, disappointed, or frustrated are more easily understood than a forgotten "Thank you" or a silent *I love you.*

Why is it we always think the other person should read between the lines and understand?

I believe it was Solomon who is quoted as saying that the greatest gift of all is an "understanding heart."

September 13, 1985

I think the world must have a heartbeat, because there are times when I know I feel its rhythm.

It was Thoreau who said: "This is a delicious evening, when the whole body is one sense, and imbibes delight through every pore."

When I feel like that, I see the world pulsating with life and beauty. I see the man with no legs striding down the hallway, smiling and swinging his arms. . . . I see my befuddled neighbor as the vibrant, gracious lady she was before her illness. . . .

Those are the thoughtful moments, too precious to share with just anyone. It is then I miss Morgan most.

Alone, I do my best to walk in step with the world.

Too bad I'm so often out of step.

September 14, 1985

I can hardly open a newspaper or listen to a newscast without being overwhelmed by the advances made in technology:

NASA's cutting through or probing into the tail of a comet with a man-made satellite is almost unbelievable, and from what I read and hear, the information that is expected to be garnered from this feat is equally almost unbelievable. . . .

And take the locating of the *Titanic,* which was made possible by the union of video and sonar in a recently developed camera. . . .

I keep wondering how all this technology—just how these miraculous developments in science will be incorporated into the quality of human life.

I was pondering this when I read an article by Cleanth Brooks, who is Gray Professor Emeritus of Rhetoric at Yale University.

Among his many degrees and honors is a B. Lit. Degree from Oxford, where he was a Rhodes scholar.

Anyway, in this article Brooks says, in essence, that a world reduced to hard scientific facts would soon become a dehumanized world in which few of us would want to live. He says that "we want to know the facts—but we crave its whole story, too—its human interest and what we call its meaning."

He cites as an example the regrettable loss of the *Titanic* and how the poet Thomas Hardy dealt with it in his poem called "Convergence of the Twain."

Brooks wrote:

Of many of the facts he makes no mention at all. He does not tell us that the date of the disaster was April 15, 1912, and that it happened on the *Titanic's* maiden voyage; that she was at 46,000 tons, the largest ship afloat; that over 1,500 lives were lost; that the ship though warned of ice ahead, was traveling at high speed; or that she was regarded as unsinkable, with double bottoms and 16 water-tight compartments.

Hardy does refer to some of these facts early in the poem but only obliquely. What caught Hardy's imagination, was that the ship and the iceberg had, with precision timing, arrived at the same spot at the same instant, just as if destiny had employed a split-second time-table for the whole affair; and he reminds his readers that while the liner was being built in the Belfast shipyard, nature had all along been preparing the mountain of ice far away on the coast of Greenland. Here are the closing stanzas of the poem:

> And as the smart ship grew
> In stature, grace and hue
> In shadowy silent distance grew the
> iceberg too.
> Alien they seemed to be;

No mortal eye could see
The intimate welding of their
                        later history,
Or sign that they were bent
By paths coincident
On being anon twin halves of
                        one august event
Till the spinner of the years
Said "Now," and each one hears
And consumption comes; and jars
                        two hemispheres.

Brooks continues, saying that we want meaning as well as information and we want wisdom.

Those two commodities, meaning and wisdom, are in short supply. "Data banks are much in vogue and they are highly useful, but they are not equipped to pay off in the currency of wisdom."

Cleanth Brooks also refers to choruses from T. S. Eliot's "The Rock":

Endless invention, endless experiment
Brings knowledge of motion but not of stillness;
Knowledge of speech, but not of silence;
Knowledge of words, and ignorance of the word . . .
Where is the wisdom we have lost in knowledge?
Where is the knowledge we have lost in information?

I wonder why, with the rush toward science in our universities, shouldn't the teaching of the humanities be emphasized to counterbalance our lopsidedness? . . . Particularly since I understand many leading corporations and medical schools, such as IBM and Johns Hopkins, are now recruiting students with liberal arts backgrounds.

There's so much to think about and philosophize over.

September 16, 1985

After talking with one of our Jewish residents this morning and noting on the calendar that today is the start of Rosh Hoshanah and later on in the month, September 25, Yom Kippur will be observed, I keep thinking what a rich heritage the Jewish people have! Too, I recall that wonderful series on TV last fall that was narrated by Abba Eban. I took notes on that documentary because I was so impressed.

According to my notes, the series chronicled over three thousand years of the Jewish people's history as it interrelated with other religions and traditions.

Major contributions have been made to Western civilization in science, literature, finance, religion, medicine, art, law. . . . whether in ethics, government, or philosophy. . . . In every social and economic development the world has felt the mark of Jewish genius.

The series was filmed in eighteen countries and on four continents. I, for one, would like to see it again!

I was very impressed as it depicted Jewish history in the context of other civilizations, ranging from Mesopotamia, Egypt, Greece, and Rome to Christian society, Moslem dominance, Europe, and America.

The documentary pointed out that there were five forces that helped ensure Jewish continuity, namely:

1. Family
2. Community
3. Religion
4. Education
5. Homeland

What wonderful concepts to have and live by.

September 19, 1985

It's twelve-thirty Thursday morning. I have been watching ABC's "45/85" program, a fascinating documentary that traced the events of world history from the end of World War II to the present. It recounted the significant moments of the past forty years.

I had thought late Wednesday afternoon that I'd jot down the happenings of this day as they affected me . . . and my feelings toward those events.

Now, after viewing and thinking about this "Night Line" program, I realize how microscopic my petty concerns were and are in relationship to world happenings.

. . . But being female and with an overabundance of human faults, I find I'm still mulling over my various emotions of this disturbing day. I guess I'm so self-centered I'm finding it hard to get off my center of gravity.

Today I was in turn hurt, no little angry, sorry, happy, disgusted, and grateful. How do I put that mixed bag of emotions into a few succinct sentences without sounding like a five-foot-two human chameleon? I don't know that I have the words.

This emotional turmoil all started because my very sore foot and leg had been bumped, pulled, and pummeled by a new, very inept aide . . . my third "inepter" since noon. I "let off steam" to Mrs. Bono, for which I was *sorry*. I was *grateful* that my competent CPA took time out from a busy day to advise me on a couple of business matters. I was *happy* that three of my long-time friends called to say hello. I become very *interested* in the "45/85" program, as it has given me much to think about today.

September 21, 1985

The autumnal equinox . . . the beginning of fall, I hope a long Missouri autumn . . . but with the chaotic weather the world has known this year, perhaps Indian summers and harvest moons will be something we'll only talk about.

Whatever comes, I love the changing seasons. I often think of them as they relate to life. I think of spring as the season of seeding or planting or *planning,* in other words. Summer to me is the season of *growing and maturing.* I see autumn as the season of *anticipation* and winter as the essence of *realization.*

I believe if one has planned well, adapted to the environment, matured during the growing years, and mellowed with the tempering and excitement of anticipation, then winter or the *realization* of one's dreams can be the most satisfying and fulfilling season of all.

September 22, 1985

Yesterday Mrs. Bono wheelchaired me through the new wing, showing me rooms she thought might be suitable for my needs. While still under construction, it's obvious the new wing will be very attractive and desirable. The rooms, however, appear smaller and there is no space comparable to the apartment-size arrangement I now occupy. There are many pluses to the new wing that may outweigh my objections to the smaller room.

At present, I'm surrounded with things I brought with me from home . . . the antique hand-carved Chinese tables that belonged to my grandmother, then to my mother, who prized them as I do . . . the antique Chinese chest . . . my Chinese oriental rugs . . . the antique hand-carved Chinese lacquer lamps . . . a coromandel screen I bought in Singapore. . . . These bits of chinoiserie, coupled with the artifacts from my travels, to Japan, Hong Kong, Malaysia, Italy, et cetera, leave me torn between sentiment and practicality.

Looking at the coromandel screen, I'm reminded of Singapore, the Chinese gentlemen who made the screen, and Raffles Hotel, particularly the Palm Garden where at dusk the hidden lights in the foliage brought out the spell of Singapore. To this day, I can almost hear the muffled sounds as they drifted in from the harbor . . . that harbor where the waters of the Indian Ocean mingled with those of the South China Sea . . . there were ships converged, berthed, and exchanged cargoes . . . teas and silks from China . . . sandalwood from India, gems and spices from Sri Lanka, timber from the jungles of Malaysia . . . goods from everywhere to everywhere.

Whenever I stopped at Raffles, I mentally peopled the verandas of the old hotel with colonels and their ladies of a bygone British empire. Even now, I can almost visualize Somerset Maugham descending the stairs to the garden—or is it Kipling?—probably Cecil Brown, just before Singapore fell to the Japanese.

I think of Singapore as it must have been in Raffles's days . . . an island of mangroves when he first saw its harbor and realized its potential.

I think of Singapore as it must have been in its colonial days, when it was a place of pink gin, officers' clubs, and genteel English ladies; I think of it when its teeming, shabby streets must have been a mixture of sights and aromas, when intrigue seemed to lurk behind every doorway . . . when the mysterious East really was the mysterious East.

Yes, and I think of Singapore as Cecil Brown must have seen it when he wrote "the incredibly stupid, but incredibly brave British pointed their guns seaward to let the Japanese infiltrate from the jungles to take over Singapore."

Today I know Singapore is a city of flower merchants . . . of buying and selling. . . . It's a tourist haven, the hotels are plush, the cuisine is superb, and the city is almost pristine clean. It may be a cold artifact, as someone once said, but I like to think of it as colorful and exciting and as the great free port . . . the great entrepôt of the Orient, as Raffles once dreamed it would be.

This bit of written rambling was all brought on by looking at the screen I hope to be able to take with me if I move.

September 23, 1985

I've decided to remain in my current apartment. After almost six years, it has become home. Aside from that, I like the "elbow room."

September 24, 1985

I must be in the minority (suppose it's the moral minority?). A young man who visits from time to time just left after vehemently defending protectionism. I kept thinking the whole time he was expounding, *Where is that wonderful self-reliance, ingenuity, and stick-to-it-iveness that made our country the leader that it is? Where is our pride of accomplishment? Aren't American people, the greatest ethnic mix in the world, capable of even more astounding innovations and improvements? Must we cry uncle every time someone takes one of our ideas and outsmarts us with it? Because of our ethnic mix, we have the ability and genius to compete with any peoples or nation of the world. Let's stop sitting back on our laurels or our duffs, if you will; let's stop sniveling. Let's roll up our sleeves and get to work. There are few heights man cannot reach if he but puts forth the effort, heart, and faith in his ability to succeed.*

September 25, 1985

Daniel Callahan of the Hastings Center, who favors continuing federal support, particularly where the elderly are concerned, says: "The crux of the matter is money, not health care. The question is Who should pay the bills?"

Continuing, he quotes an elderly American as follows: "We don't like to take money from our kids. . . . They don't like giving us money either . . . so we all sign a political contract. . . . The young people give money to the government. . . . . I get money from the government. That way we both get mad at the government and keep on loving each other."

Funny and sad, but how true!

September 26, 1985

As I've grown older, I find I don't require as much sleep as I once did. If I awaken in the middle of the night, as I often do, I turn on (very softly, of course) CBS's "Nightwatch" program, which always has something interesting, entertaining, informative, or, as was the case this morning, very beautiful.

CBS's program, "Prayer in Song," was a rerun featuring Jan Pierce. His beautiful voice caught all the poignancy, pathos, and hope of the Hebrew songs he sang to commemorate Yom Kippur. I'm told Pierce's faith was as fine and beautiful as his voice.

I'm certain I, a Gentile, was as touched and moved as any Jew who listened to the words and music.

September 29, 1985

It was my privilege to make several buying trips to Japan when I was employed by SBF. That beautiful little island country always fascinated me. While I still correspond on occasion with a couple of Japanese friends I made on those trips, I confess I'm among the many Americans who do not really understand the Japanese mind or the psychology that "makes it tick."

Reading the article "Lost Samurai" in *Harpers*, by Henry Scott Stokes, made me realize all the more what is meant by "loss of face" and how deeply that hurts those tradition-bound people and the damage that loss does to the Japanese psyche.

Stokes first went to Japan as a young correspondent for the London *Financial Times.* After a two-year stint, he returned to London completely frustrated by his inability to understand the Japanese mind. After a year, he returned to Japan as a correspondent for the *London Times.* Later he was Tokyo Bureau chief for the *New York Times.*

On his first trip, Stokes thought all he had to do was "eat a little sushi, go to the Noh Theatre, meet a geisha or two, then return to England as a full-fledged Japan Hand . . . ready to interpret the meaning of the New Asia to a breathless West."

For all his well-meaning efforts, he was "unable to make contact with the reality of Japanese life."

After spending the year in England, he returned to Japan determined to learn the language, speak it fluently, and get to the bottom of the Japanese enigma. It was then he met and learned to know and admire the noted novelist Yukio Mishima, who later committed hara-kiri as a protest against the emperor for surrendering to the Americans and for Japan's subsequent bitter loss of face in military defeat.

Stokes contends Japan's postwar prosperity is a "mere triviality. . . . Its vast wealth is minimal compensation for the hideous humiliation of the American Occupation . . . and the American-Way-of-Life the Japanese have affected in the years since 1945."

In a way Mishima's suicide, according to Stokes, represented a "Nobility of Failure" or a "Spiritual Coup d'etat."

In substance Stokes closes his article saying it's hard not to wonder if an atomic Japan might in the end choose the evil beauty of mass destruction. His concluding frightening and heart-breaking comment is. "I am sure of this . . . the world is in enough trouble as it is without adding to its infinite complications the terrifying prospect of a suicidal nuclear-armed Japan."

September 30, 1985

Why is it that healthy, able-bodied people with good arms, legs, and eyesight can't walk by a wheelchair without blundering into it or bumping it in some manner?

This usually happens to me when I'm at the dinner table, just in the process of lifting a forkful of some food or ready to take a sip of beverage, when, voilà, it's all over the front of me.

Annoyed? No! Angry? Yes! All of which makes me think of the book *Don't Get Mad—Get Even.*

What should I do in this case? Throw the first thing I can reach on the table? That's an idea! Perhaps if the careless person who jolted me found a plate of spaghetti or a glob of chocolate pudding dripping from his or her shoulder, that person might be more circumspect when my wheelchair comes into view.

P.S. I've just sent two blouses to the dry cleaner's.

October 2, 1985

Yesterday, despite my wheelchair bumps, was generally a day of pleasant happenings for me.

Gerry B—— and "Deeter" stopped by. . . . Deeter brought me a beautiful, blossoming gardenia plant. It's really quite magnificent and I spent much of last evening and most of today sniffing and admiring and being completely enthralled by its beauty.

Trina D——, one of COTG's very caring aides, added to my enjoyment by bringing her perky little schnauzer, Bridget, in to see me. Loving animals as I do, dogs in particular, I was happy to pet and cuddle Bridget.

I wish it were possible for me to keep a "pet of my very own" here at the nursing home.

October 3, 1985

I'm still looking for a private duty nurse aide. I ran an ad again yesterday. The response to my previous ad had not been too good. One woman wanted to know if I wouldn't adjust my required hours to fit her free time. Another wanted more than twice the going rate for nurse aides. Two others were college students whose classes conflicted with my needed hours. Perhaps yesterday's ad will bring better results. I'm hoping!

And people still talk about unemployment. They can't be too hungry or too ambitious.

October 5, 1985

Sometimes I wonder about me . . . the idleness or restlessness of my curiosity . . . the great variety of subjects that interest me. Am I lacking in purpose? Is my mind nothing more than a vagabond that takes pleasure in roaming the pathways of literature, music, philosophy, even the unknown boundaries of science and/or the vagaries of human nature?

Sadly, I'm not proficient in anything. I'm a dabbler into anything that catches my interest. If my interest is sufficiently aroused, I pursue that subject, seeking its history, background, the whys and wherefores of it. For example, if I look up a word or name in a dictionary or encyclopedia—almost anything will trigger my research—I then find that one word or name leads to another and that starts me digging . . . only to bring up another word, name, or association. It's unending. I have the desire to continue . . . . to keep on searching, reading, and absorbing . . . but I'm not quite as strong physically as I once was and I find myself tiring much sooner than I'd like. I'm determined, however, to build up my strength and endurance. Why, yesterday I walked to the dining room (something I haven't done in three years), sat in a regular dining chair, enjoyed luncheon, and walked back to my room. I was tired, very tired, but I'm going to do it again and again. Who knows? Perhaps someday I'll be able to take that walk all by myself. Now I need a steel leg brace, a quad cane, and someone walking alongside of me (in the event I should lose my balance.)

There's always tomorrow! In the interim, I'll continue creating an interesting world of my own.

October 6,1 985

I've been leafing through N-M's *Christmas 1985,* that extravaganza of retail catalogues; this is the twenty-fifth year of Nieman-Marcus's legendary his and her gifts. As usual, they are breathtaking in imagination, price, and, as in the case this year, beauty.

I merely paused over this year's magnificent pair of yellow diamonds . . . cut from a single rough and priced at $2 million . . . but I was stopped, not only to admire but to reminisce when I turned to the page containing an exquisite Faberge enamel.

It was in the late forties or early fifties. I was a jewelry buyer at the time and was in New York on a buying trip when Maurice S. Jelenko, general merchandise manager of SBF, called me and asked if I'd meet him at the Russian Gift Shop on Fifth Avenue. It was located just north of the old Savoy Plaza, where I was stopping. The shop was managed or owned by a gentleman by the name of Schaeffer, if I remember correctly.

I met Mr. Jay (as most of his underlings called him) as requested, and was introduced to Mr. Schaeffer, who took us back to the sanctum sanctorus, a room containing a huge wall safe.

Because Mr. Jay thought I should see what some world famous jewelry looked like at close range, I was shown a diamond necklace that supposedly once belonged to Catherine the Great. I was impressed, of course, but not as much as when Mr. Schaeffer told me the story of Carl Faberge, court jeweler to the Russian czars . . . and then handed me a small three-inch exquisitely enameled box made by Faberge. He asked me to guess the price.

Knowing it had to be expensive, I thought I'd guess high and hesitatingly said "Seventy-five hundred dollars?"

"No," Mr. Schaeffer answered. "It's priced at sixteen thousand." I thought the price astronomical then. After looking at N-M's enameled oval box two and a half by two and three sixteenths by one inch priced at two hundred thousand dollars, I can't help wondering what that little three-inch box, which I so lovingly held in my hands, would be worth today? Not as much as my memories, I'll wager.

October 11, 1985

COTG took several interested residents for a tour last Monday to see the renovated Union Station. To me it was an exhilarating experience. I found it a stimulating day . . . but an exhausting one. I had sat in my wheelchair from 8: 00 A.M. until 5: 00 P.M. and was dog-tired when I wheeled myself back to my room.

Were I ambulatory, I'd take a room at the Omni International for a few days and spend my time looking into every corner of the renovation.

I'd spend a few hours in the grand hall, just looking and admiring; I'd climb the stairways, touch some of the grill work, and even touch some of the repainted baggage trucks. I'd try to figure out all by myself where Fred Harvey's was once located, where the stationmaster's office, the huge newsstand, the baggage room . . . where everything I still remember was once located.

I can still visualize the milling crowds and the jammed waiting room concourse during and following World War II. That old station was the start and ending of so many of my buying trips. One such trip I remember in particular. It was shortly after the end of the war . . . sometime in the late forties.

I was by then using planes more often than trains. On this trip I was flying in from New York. The plane was filled with servicemen. There were only three women aboard . . . a young teenage wife returning to her family after visiting her army husband stationed in the east, an elderly white-haired lady who was to be met by her son in St. Louis, and I, returning home from a buying trip. For some reason, we couldn't land in St. Louis and were forced to go on to Kansas City. There in the old terminal, with the other two women, who had gravitated to me, I learned there were no planes available to get us to St. Louis but that we might be able to get a "milk-run" that was leaving within the hour. I knew we'd have to hurry and that we could buy our tickets on the train. I asked if the other two women wanted to come with me. They did. I managed to reach Morgan by phone and asked if he'd call the other two families, explaining to them what had happened and when we might be expected to arrive in St. Louis by train.

Getting to the Kansas City Union Station was not too much of a "time" problem in those days, as that was long before the new KC airport had been built on the outskirts.

Everything went well; we three women took a cab to the station, boarded the train, and were arranging with the conductor to buy our tickets when the young wife burst into tears, explaining that she had no money. I bought her ticket and told her not to worry. The elderly lady then said that she had enough money but would need my help in getting to it. She asked if I'd come with her to the washroom. The conductor, longsuffering, I suspect, agreed to wait. In the washroom I helped milady unpin numerous five-dollar bills "safety-pinned" to her corset and other undergarments.

It was a milk-run train with stops every few miles, but we finally arrived in St. Louis, where we were met by our families. The plane ride from New York to St. Louis was a first flight for the elderly lady, and the train ride from Kansas City to St. Louis was a first for the young wife.

I later received very gracious thank you notes. . . . The son who met his mother turned out to be head of OPA in St. Louis at the time and was very grateful for my shepherding of his mother.

The girl's family was equally grateful and enclosed a check for her train fare with their gracious note.

October 15, 1985

Today was a very happy day. Meredith Patton of Princeton, New Jersey, visiting her father in St. Louis, took time out to spend some time with me this afternoon. Much as I appreciated her gift, I didn't need the box of chocolates to remind me of what a thoughtful lady she is. After she left, Kenny W—— called. His cheery hellos are always treasured.

In the evening, Emily B—— spent a couple of hours with me. She is delightful company. She bought me a plant spray to mist the beautiful gardenia plant Deeter gave me.

So much pleasant attention and all in one day. Suspect I'll go to sleep tonight in a holiday mood.

October 16, 1985

I've been sorting through some old pictures of Echo Valley, and I keep asking myself why I've had no desire to go back to see it. I guess I'm a coward. . . . I think I don't want to see it as it might be today. I had the feeling at the time I sold Echo Valley that the purchaser was a developer and promoter. I was assured otherwise, but I had an uneasy feeling that those beautiful tree-laden acres would be plotted and sold in one half and one-acre increments.

I choose now and apparently chose unconsciously then to always remember it as it was. In my reverie, I see it as the lovely place Morgan and I planned as our retirement home.

I've learned to break with the past . . . but I know I'll always cherish its memories.

October 17, 1985

Yesterday the baseball Cardinals clinched the National League playoff series by defeating the Los Angeles Dodgers. The Kansas City Royals defeated the Toronto Blue Jays for the American League. Now it will become a Missouri World Series battle between St. Louis and Kansas City.

The last time the National and American League winners fought it out in Missouri was in 1944, when the St. Louis Cards and the St. Louis Browns faced each other.

Morgan and I and some of our friends attended two or three of these games. Then I was a Brownie fan, probably because I tend to always favor the underdog.

I'm certain many St. Louisans remember the *Post Dispatch* "Weatherbird," that clever daily cartoon with its often amusing comments. The following comment, which I've probably garbled, comes to mind because it hurt my Brownie sentiments. "St. Louis, first in shoes, first in booze and last in the American League."

Well, it went something like that.

October 19, 1985

I was watching the Missouri-Nebraska football game today when one of the aides, who brought me fresh towels, said, "I didn't know you liked football. I suppose you went to Mizzou."

I replied that I hadn't attended the University of Missouri but that I like college football, in fact, preferring it to professional football because of its excitement and color, the marching bands, et cetera. After the aide left, I realized why I had been switching back and forth on TV channels to watch the play and get the scores of specific games.

I was interested in the Missouri-Nebraska game because my father had gone to the University of Nebraska and my paternal grandfather had been one of the trustees of that university. Too, my mother, father, and I were all born in Nebraska. I was interested in the Iowa-Michigan game because of their #1 and #2 ratings this year. It was an exciting game!

As for the Ohio State–Purdue game, I kept tuning in to that game because of my attachment for Ohio State. Morgan had gone to college there and I had a brief stint there during my sophomore year, when I left Northwestern for a few months to be nearer Dayton and my ailing mother.

No doubt my very special feelings for Ohio State go back to my freshman year at Northwestern, when I was the guest of the Ohio State football team at a musical comedy in Chicago.

This all come about because Ohio State was playing Northwestern in Evanston. A young man from Dayton by the name of Vernie Reboulet was on the Ohio State squad. Vernie and I had attended the same high school (Stivers) in Dayton. We had dated off and on during those halcyon days. I don't know how Vernie managed it, but Dr. Wills, who was the Ohio State coach at the time, arranged for me to be picked up in Evanston by cab and driven to Chicago, where I joined the lads from Ohio State to see the musical comedy *Good News* before the team took the midnight train back to Columbus.

I don't recall too much about the comedy except for two memorable songs, "Varsity Drag" and "The Best Things in Life Are Free."

Following the show I was put in a cab, as Vernie and the team stood waving good-bye. I was taken back to Evanston and the Freshman Campus View House on Sheridan Road, where I lived my first year at Northwestern. I know I was the most excited and happiest little co-ed on campus. . . . That was 1928 . . . fifty-seven years ago, and I still enjoy college football.

October 22, 1985

Eight of us "inmates" were taken to Powell Hall last evening to hear Woody Herman. Apparently I was the only one who really enjoyed his music. The others, for the most part, thought his orchestra was too loud and brassy. It seemed loud to me, too. I thought a bit more muting would have helped, but I still enjoyed his jazz musicianship. Perhaps that appreciation stems from the fact that long ago

I had danced to his music and even attended his Carnegie Hall concert held sometime in the mid- or late forties. It was for this concert that Igor Stravinsky wrote his only work for a Jazz orchestra . . . *The Ebony Concerto.*

Richard Stoltzman, well-know classical clarinetist, was guest artist last evening. He played the concerto beautifully, I thought. Of course among the selections played by the orchestra during the evening were "The Woodchoppers' Ball" and "Blue Flame," the Herman theme song. I liked it all.

October 23, 1985

I keep a small two-drawer file in my room. Because it's difficult for me to do any filing from my wheelchair. I often ask others to file papers for me. I'm frequently amazed not only at *what* is filed but *where* it is filed.

Today I was looking for an appraisal and came up with an article on Caswell-Massey, the oldest apothecary shop and perfumer in the United States.

Rereading the article, by John Berendt and published in *Cosmopolitan* Magazine, I was reminded of the pleasure I had in working with this firm when I merchandised the cosmetic and drug departments of SBF. We put in Caswell-Massey products in a small exclusive shop at SBF's Westroads Store.

What happened to the shop after SBF changed ownership I do not know. Because there's no longer a C-M shop at Westroads, I order their products from the New York store. At present, I have soap, cologne, potpourri, and a potpourri oil on order.

But more about that unique shop at the corner of Lexington Avenue and 48th Street. In the words of Berendt; "To go to C-M is to find yourself in an emporium for the pampered self . . . at a PX for voluptuaries with a taste for the past."

When I knew C-M, it was owned by Ralph and Milton Taylor. It may still be. I suspect it is . . . or is being run by some member of the family who has great respect for quality and tradition.

Leafing through their catalog to me is more fun than reading a novel. Everything is stocked, from lavender smelling salts and potpourris to bear grease and the greatest selection of soaps I've ever heard of or known. There's seaweed soap, tomato, lettuce, soapless soap, even five kinds of soap from India, to name a few. I often buy their sandalwood soap, as well as their famous almond and cold cream soap.

Once this firm, dating back to 1752, sold leeches at $4.50 each.

Even today you can buy curved and straight mustache scissors . . . and, of course, mustache combs, brushes, and waxes. These are but a few of the myriad of items difficult to find elsewhere.

According to Berendt, Jacqueline Onassis and John Denver are among the many celebrities who buy from C-M. The cologne made for George Washington is still made and sold, as is the face cream once made for and used by Sarah Bernhardt.

It's the most fascinating shop I know, and I've loved the firm ever since I heard the Taylors closed down their whole line of whale-oil soaps when they learned whales were becoming extinct.

October 26, 1985

As I looked around COTG this morning, I wondered, as I often to, what makes some people give up and others keep on keeping on. I particularly noticed two residents.

When they first came here, both were physically handicapped, but alert, socially gracious, interesting persons to talk with and be around. Today one appears to be angry at the world and sour on everyone in it. The other is hardly aware he's living and apparently couldn't care less.

What causes a person to give up? Is it illness? Loneliness? Lack of family support? Loss of self-esteem? Lack of motivation? Or the ever-present enervating influence of nursing home associates who are debilitated?

And what motivates those of us who keep on keeping on? Is it the right combination of genes and early environment?

I believe I'm a "keeper-on." Not that there aren't times when I feel life has shortchanged me . . . when I silently cry, sometimes not so silently, because I can hear me even if no one else does. It is then I'd like to sit in the middle of the floor and pound my heels (if I could physically) and tell anyone who tries to interrupt my childish tantrum to go to hell. Perhaps it's my fighting back that keeps me going.

Whatever it is, something inside me (perhaps that still, small voice) tells me to stop thinking of myself and start practicing what I so boringly preach.

It is then I remember I only have myself to look after. Others have greater responsibilities. There's Esther W——, for example, who for as long as I can remember (and we've been friends for forty-five years) has looked after a disturbed brother (only five years younger than she) who has never worked a day in his life. Esther has been his sole support financially, spiritually, emotionally, intellectually, and in every other way you can think of, ever since their parents died, almost fifty years ago. I don't have the nerve to complain! Or not to keep on keeping on.

October 27, 1985

Tonight I was embarrassed for the Cardinals . . . not because they lost the World Series, but because they were not good losers. No one likes to lose, but some people take defeat better than others. I kept hoping all through the game that the Cards would handle their rout with at least some degree of dignity. . . . Unfortunately, they didn't.

October 29, 1985

St. Louisans celebrated the twentieth anniversary of their gleaming stainless steel Gateway Arch last weekend

According to its history, the arch began as a dream in the mind of a civic-minded St. Louisan named Luther Ely Smith. That was in 1933, more than three decades before the arch was topped-out on October 28, 1965.

Today the arch is a not only monument to the dream and tenacity of Luther Ely Smith, but a standing symbol of Eero Saarinen's genius as an architect and the engineering sophistication of the McDonald Construction Company of St. Louis and subcontractor Pittsburgh–Des Moines Steel Company of Pittsburgh.

Quoting the *Globe-Democrat* of October 19–20, Charles E. Caspari, current present of the Jefferson National Expansion Association, said:

> We didn't know what his [Smith's] vision was, but we knew it was going to be something great. We would be satisfied with nothing else.
>
> The entire concept, full of exciting possibilities for actual achievement, is a work of genius and the memorial structure is of that high order which will rank it among the nation's greatest monuments.

Almost insurmountable obstacles had to be overcome before the 630 foot stainless steel arch became a reality and one of the nation's outstanding tourist attractions.

Jerry L. Schober, superintendent of the Jefferson National Expansion Memorial, is quoted as saying, "The arch didn't become a reality by people giving up."

November 1, 1985

This is one of those days (as was yesterday) when I should have stood in bed. . . . At least I think I'd be able to breathe more easily. . . . I'm sure there's a reason for my sinuses performing as they are. . . . Humidity? Barometric pressure? Allergy index? All brought on by the whiplash of tropical storm Juan? I don't know—I just know my head feels like a stuffed cabbage, my throat is raw, and my breathing is as labored-sounding as Jack Benny's Maxwell when it revved up on the radio show of long ago.

To take my mind off my uncomfortable physical condition, I've been listening to all the news programs I can find, everyone's comments regarding the Russian lad some thought wanted to seek asylum in the United States, others thought not, Reagan's new and/or counterproposals for the Geneva arms control meetings, the forthcoming summit, et cetera, et cetera.

While there's certainly no similarity, I couldn't help but be reminded of the time I interviewed two Russians. That was in the mid- or late thirties, and I was Women's Page editor of the *Dayton Journal-Herald* at the time. When I met Baron and Baroness Charles Wrangell, they were representing the Helena Rubenstein cosmetic line. They, rather she, Countess Leda Wrangell, was appearing at the Rike Kumler Company, where I interviewed them. Countess Wrangell was the former Leda Utgoff, widow of well-known Russian ace of World War I, Victor Utgoff. Baron Wrangell was a member of the family after whom Wrangell Island was named. Also, he was a former member of the Corps des Pages to the last Russian czar, Nicholas.

Accepting my invitation, the Wrangells spent a couple of evenings at my home. During their week's stay in Dayton, they told me many fascinating things about their lives. Both had escaped Russia during the Bolshevik revolution.

The Utgoffs, with their two sons, had made their way to the United States via Sebastapol and London. During that travail, many of their experiences were harrowing. Once in the States, Victor joined the Coast Guard. He was later killed in a plane accident and was buried in Arlington Cemetery.

Several years later, Leda met Baron Wrangell and they were married.

For some time following their visit to Dayton, we kept in touch. Today I only have a yellowed graduation announcement from Annapolis telling me of the graduation of Leda's older son, Vladim.

Oh, yes, and somewhere in my file is a photostat of some of the Russian émigrés, sent to me by Baron Wrangell.

The Wrangells were a striking and charming couple. She was a very beautiful woman.

November 4, 1985

I wonder what the Mad Hatter, the Duchess, and Tweedledum said when the original boxwood blocks used in illustrating their antics were recently found in a vault of the Coventry Garden branch of London's National Westminster Bank.

An executive of MacMillan Publishers, in making a routine check of the company's materials, found a black box labeled "Alice," "Wonderland," and "Looking Glass." The box was broken into to reveal the long forgotten blocks.

Lewis Carroll, whose real name was Charles Ludgwidge Dodgson, was a mathematics don at Oxford and had commissioned and paid John Tenniel (later called Sir John), an illustrator, to make the drawings for his "Alice" books. Tenniel received 138 pounds for the *Wonderland* sketches. That was four pounds less than Carroll paid the engravers.

According to the article I read in the *Monitor*, both Carroll and Tenniel were perfectionists and the very first edition of *Alice* was withdrawn because of their dissatisfaction with the printing. Only twenty copies of this edition are supposed to have survived. Subsequent editions met their standards. However, the wood blocks have never been used *directly* since. Instead, durable metal electroplates were made (a practice of the time) from the blocks and used for the continuous flow of editions since.

A MacMillan spokesman said, "No commercial edition of the prints has ever been published, so far as I know, from the wood blocks."

MacMillan now plans to use the blocks in an exclusive and limited edition of individual prints that will be available in September or October of 1986: "The edition will be small, probably only 200 sets, and expensive."

I didn't fall down a rabbit hole, but I can almost see the Cheshire Cat grinning and nodding his head at the March Hare—or is that the Mock Turtle?

November 7, 1985

Hearing about the Picasso exhibit currently taking place in Montreal, I'm reminded of Victor Ganz and what he did with the five major Picassos he owned.

I knew Victor Ganz years ago, when I was a fashion jewelry buyer and he was the head of D. Lisner Company of New York, a costume jewelry house. As I recall, his interest in Picasso had started years before when he began collecting small Picasso sketches.

Somewhere in my small but bursting-at-its-seams file, there's an article about Victor Ganz and his Picassos. I'll ask an aide to help me find it. I do remember, however, that using a sitting room in his Fifth Avenue apartment, he arranged with Robsjohn-Giddings to create a background for the five major paintings he owned. These paintings were five of the fifteen studies made by Picasso of the well-known Delacroix painting *Women of Algiers.*

. . . Found the June 1960 *Vogue* Magazine article that describes this made-to-order room as follows: "The room has the controlled airiness of a latticed window, a spindled door, and grey-white color all over as a backdrop. The walls, ceilings, vinyl floor, upholstery, Moroccan tables, Indian lamps and ancient wares collected especially for the room quietly evoke the Delacroix-Picasso oriental theme."

Critics claimed the quiet room was the perfect setting for the five colorful, vibrant Picasso studies.

Reading on, I learned that at the time of the *Vogue* article, one of the Ganz-owned paintings was on exhibition at the Tate Gallery in London.

According to my reference books, Eugene Delacroix was an "elegant master of the Romantic movement in France." In 1832 he spent six months in Morocco, Tangiers, and Algeria, then a newly acquired French possession. From the sketches made on this sojourn came his famous 1834 painting, *Women of Algiers*, which is now hanging in the Louvre.

November 9, 1985

Mickie F—— frequently comes to my room after dinner. We either listen to music or a TV program or I read aloud to her or we just sit and talk.

Last evening we chose to chat. During our random conversation, the subject of schools and teachers came up. Mickie reminisced about the small country one-room school she attended in Iowa and the caring, competent teacher who had laid the groundwork academically for Mickie to continue on in high school and college.

Long after Mickie left, my thoughts roamed back to my school days and those teachers who had left lasting impressions on me. There were many such teachers, but the one who comes to mind most often was a short, dynamic Hungarian by the name of Hosco at the University of Dayton law school. I, the only girl in the school at the time, was in one of his classes on torts. If any one of us, when called upon to brief a case, begged or started wandering all over the lot in reaching the point, we were certain to be interrupted with, "Vwher iss my lefft ear?"

Raising his right arm and circling it over his head, he'd laboriously point to his left ear and say, "Ach, here iss my lefft ear!"

To this day whenever I see someone incompetently handling a job or hear someone "beating around the bush" in trying to explain something, I immediately think, *Vwher iss my left ear?*

At the time I was in one of Dr. Hosco's classes, the following story was told about him. Whether it was true or not, I do not know, but observing Hosco at the time and remembering him so vividly since, I can well believe the story was true.

Dr. Hosco, so the story went, had been a prominent attorney in Budapest before coming to this country. One day a member of the Hungarian aristocracy came to him, explaining that a son, who worked in a bank, had absconded with what would be fifty thousand in U.S. currency. The young man had squandered the money, then became scared and the night before had gone to his father beseeching his help.

The father told Hosco the family would sell land and any or all possessions to make restitution. Was there any way Hosco could save the family from disgrace?

Dr. Hosco asked that the young man be sent to see him at once. This was done and Hosco is supposed to have asked him if he could easily appropriate another fifty thousand dollars from the bank. If so, he was to do it immediately and bring the money, securities or whatever was negotiable to Hosco. The young man complied and Hosco then marched the young man with the money to the bank officials, telling them that the boy, scion of a fine old Hungarian family, had stolen one hundred thousand dollars from the bank, was contrite and frightened, but could return fifty thousand dollars at once. The balance would be raised by the family selling land, silver plate, heirlooms, or whatever it took to pay back the bank in full.

According to the story, Hosco's proposition was accepted, the bank was paid, the son went free, and the family honor remained intact.

As far as I know, the story may still be making the rounds in the corridors of the University of Dayton.

Still November 9, 1985
I've often said I'd never die of anything serious; it would be just out-and-out frustration . . . trying to do something physically that my handicap prevents me from accomplishing.

At present, I'm looking around my room. . . . Over there is a drawer I can't quite close, a stack of magazines that needs to be sorted, some given away, others to be thrown out, books I can't put back in the bookcases, linen that should be sent to the laundry, chest drawers that need to be straightened and rearranged. Too, I should go through my closet and give away or pitch out half that's there.

So far, applicants for private duty nursing have been few and I've run three ads. Mrs. Bono who has been looking at and screening applicants for me, too, has found no one so far she feels I should consider or interview.

Doesn't anyone want to work anymore?

November 10, 1985
I was leafing through a catalog on Russian lacquer boxes yesterday and was reminded of the Russian lacquer box I own. I didn't know where it was at the moment but thought it might be tucked back on one of my bookshelves. When Emily B—— visited me last evening, I asked if she'd look for it. She did and found it.

My box is three and seven-eights by two and three-quarters by one inch and is a pretty little thing. The outside is black with a small, colorful floral design on the top. The inside is red. On the bottom of the box is inscribed: MADE IN USSR BD 168.

I know my box isn't valuable as compared to those listed in the catalog, which sell for hundreds of dollars. I probably only paid a few dollars for mine. I remember thinking at the time it was quite inexpensive.

The story of the enamel boxes has always fascinated me. According to their history, *all Russian enamel boxes* are crafted in a tiny area some three hundred kilometers northwest of Moscow. In this area are the villages of Mystera, Kholui, Fedoskino, and Palekh. Each village has its own style and favorite subjects for decoration, fairy tales, village scenes, landscapes, bouquets, et cetera.

The villagers work together to create their unique designs, using methods that have been passed on for generations. Some cut cardboard to size, cover it with paste, press it in a mold to dry, then dip it in linseed oil. After that, the carpenters take over. They plane and sand the forms. They apply putty made by hand to each box and pumice it for smoothness, so that the painters can readily coat each box with lacquer, the outside in black, the inside in red. After an additional coat of lacquer is applied, the box is sent to the artist.

The artist draws an outline of the desired decoration, paints it in with zinc white, and covers it with colors, which are egg-emulsion tempora, made fresh in extremely small quantities. Gold leaf is then applied and burnished with a wolf's tooth. All artists make their own brushes from squirrel hair and paint their detailed designs with the aid of a magnifying glass. Finally, the artist signs the box and adds the title and registration number and the name of his village. Although different boxes may share the same theme, every box is individual in its execution.

After reviewing the history of this art, I wonder if my little box isn't an orphan. Even so, I love it . . . as orphans are so often loved. On second thought, it may not be an orphan. . . .

November 13, 1985

Paraphrasing an old song, "Wrap Your Troubles in Dreams," *I wrapped my memories in remembered music* last evening when I joined seven other residents and three staff members to enjoy Larry Elgart and His Hooked on Swing Orchestra at Powell Hall.

The whole evening was reminiscent of the Big Band era that Morgan and I danced through. The Elgart orchestra played many of the theme songs and music made famous by the Big Bands of the forties and fifties. What is more, Elgart gave credit to other bands and musicians *and* he gave credit to the arrangers, such as Johnson and Murtaugh.

I'm afraid I was a bit misty-eyed when songs such as "String of Pearls" and "In the Mood" were played.

November 14, 1985

I'm an Anglophile . . . have been for as long as I can remember . . . or as long as I had any comprehension of the dimension of world history but I'm glad the Prince and Princess of Wales are on their way home. . . .

Not that most Americans didn't enjoy their visit. They did!

Not that the British haven't given us much. They have!

Not that the U.S. hasn't been generous in appreciation. It has! And most Britishers acknowledge that!

And granted the royal couple is charming, then why, with this existing mutual respect, just why do some Americans, yes, and some members of the media "go gushy ga-ga" over "his" impeccable grooming and "her" beautiful gowns?

Personally, I'd like to see us stress those things, really meaningful things, that we have given to each other and the world.

For example, I'm thinking of Greenwich Mean Time, the gift that English resourcefulness gave the world, "timing" it and us for generations. Now, Greenwich time is depending on an American satellite for its millionth of a second accuracy. American ingenuity and space technology were the reciprocal gifts of the U.S.

I like to think of our two countries curtsying to each other for things of that sort . . . or am I being stuffy?

November 18, 1985

They were quarreling outside my door, and I couldn't help but hear Annie shouting, "Shut up, Joe!"

Joe yelled back, "I don't have to shut up. I can talk when I want to."

Annie answered, "That may be, but shut up when you talk to me."

November 19, 1985

The eyes, ears, and prayers of the world are centered on Geneva today.

I watched (on TV, of course) President Reagan and Secretary General Gorbachev shaking hands this morning before entering the lakeside chateau where they spent an hour talking before their first formal meeting.

I may be an incurable optimist, but I believe the forthcoming summit talks will be the *start* of paving the way or building that longed-for bridge between our two countries.

. . . And I'm glad there's a news blackout. It should prevent some of the media speculation and often distortion of facts. I have enough faith to wait . . . and believe that when the two leaders make a joint or separate statement, the news will be upbeat and progress indicated.

November 21, 1985

Apparently the chemistry was right . . . at least not incompatible. To me, the joint statement made by Reagan and Gorbachev pointed to better understanding between the two leaders and hopefully the *START* of a better relationship between our two countries. It will take time, increased understanding, and mutual trust to develop a substantive arms reduction program . . . or so it seems to me.

* * *

Sometimes I wonder if the nurse aides, nurses, and above all supervisors realize how very *stressful* it is to an ill, handicapped, or infirm resident to have the seemingly constant change of personnel that greets us on most of the shifts.

I realize from my own experience in trying to find a competent aide how difficult it must be to staff a nursing facility or even a hospital where the infirm, sick, and crotchety must be handled. Yet there are two sides to that coin and for every obnoxious oldster there's an inept know-it-all young aide. I've arrived at the point where I hate to see my door open and a new face appear. I cringe, get uptight, and often unjustifiably think, *Oh, no! Not another one to try to tell how to transfer me, how not to pull my paralyzed arm or hit my very tender foot against the side of the bed, chair, tub, or even wall.* I must admit sometimes the aide misses the wall, but seldom the side of the whirlpool tub. Then there's my stiff knee, which most new aides try to bend by "pump-handling" my leg, which only makes my leg and foot more rigid. It is then the muscles in my leg start to spasm and I become that unreasonable old lady on 300 hall who demands "that someone assist me who knows what she's doing."

November 22, 1985

I was told a story today that is probably as old as I am, but I'd never heard it before and it amused me. I'm no storyteller, but the tale went something like this:

It seems the Creator, when He'd finished making man, told him he'd given him twenty years for a good, healthy sex life. Man objected, saying he deserved more time. The Creator said He'd think the matter over, but at the moment He had to get on with making the monkey.

When he'd finished, the Creator told the monkey He'd give him twenty years to enjoy a healthy sex life, too. The monkey answered saying that was too much time; he only needed ten years. Upon hearing that, man asked if he might have the other ten years. The Creator nodded yes, then started at once to fashion the lion. While working, He told the lion he too would be given twenty years to enjoy a healthy sex life. The lion demurred, saying twenty years was much too long, but that he'd like ten years. Man was delighted and asked if he might have the remaining ten years. The Creator agreed and hurried to make the donkey, to whom He gave twenty years to enjoy a healthy sex life. Like the lion and the monkey, the donkey told the Creator that ten years would be sufficient. The Creator agreed and as the story goes, that is how or why man has twenty years to enjoy a normal, healthy sex life, ten years to monkey around, ten years of lying about it, and ten years to make a jackass of himself.

30

Using-30-to end my story is a throwback to my newspaper days when-thirty-was then used by all reporters to let the typesetters in the composing room know that was the end of the article, story, or bit of copy.

I wonder if that is the practice today . . . or is that as outmoded as highbutton shoes and two-parent households?

149

November 23, 1985

If spoken, I'm sure my silent conjecturing about space, infinity, the "Big Bang" time, "Black Holes," galaxies, et cetera, would make some people think I'm a charter member of the lunatic fringe. Of course, I don't think I am, but then who does when he's a bit "wacky" according to some standards?

The more I read, the more convinced I am, in my own mind, that there's no conflict between science and religion. That super-power (as I call it) whose accomplishments are beyond human du-plication, even human comprehension, is to me God, and my faith is centered around the thought that with God nothing is impossible.

If we humans but had the courage, stick-to-it-iveness, and *faith* to believe, how much happier we'd be.

November 26, 1985

Forty-eight years ago today on November 26, 1937, Morgan and I were married. I lost him on February 26, 1978, just three months to the day after our fortieth wedding anniversary.

Now, as then, he's in my heart. Today he's not only in my heart but in my memories.

That love and those memories have kept the nursing home walls from closing in on me.

Thanksgiving, November 28, 1985

It has been a beautiful day. Many of my friends and I touched base. Some of those friendships go back to 1940, when Morgan and I first came to St. Louis. Esther, Sally, Nell, Marge, Gerry, and I all exchanged greetings and good wishes and thanked the power that is for all the blessings that have come our way. Jim Ream, my cousin's son who's with NASA in Florida, wasn't too busy to call me. What a thoughtful and fine young man he is.

The Thanksgiving dinner at COTG was excellent as always, and Mrs. Bono was her usual charming self.

December 4, 1985

Today marks my sixth year at Clayton-on-the-Green. It took me a long, agonizing time to make the adjustment from the life I once knew to the necessary life-style of a nursing home.

At first I didn't know if I would or could adapt. And I'm certain

I must have been the proverbial "pain in the neck" to everyone here for too long a time after my arrival. I literally hated the very idea of a nursing home.

Finally, I came to my senses and realized I'd only destroy myself if I let feelings of frustration, resentment, and anger take over. I guess I had too much pride, willpower, and self-confidence to be defeated by a stroke and subsequent nursing home life.

Anyway, today I've managed to climb over most of the self-imposed hurdles that blocked my progress. More important, I can live with myself . . . . the standards I set for myself and my conscience. I even like living at COTG most of the time.

December 7, 1985

The formal opening this week of COTG's new wing has been hectic and stressful for residents and staff alike. The dedicated staff has worked long hours training new personnel, getting acquainted with and making comfortable the new incoming residents, and re-locating and placating present residents who resisted new seating arrangements in the enlarged dining room.

The occasional inadvertent setting off the alarm system and work-men cutting into the wrong electrical or water lines only added spice to work-filled days, or so the weary staff said.

The other evening at dinner, I asked a new waitress for a glass of water. Her answer was, "I'm not in charge of that, babe, but I'll see what I can do." Yes, eventually she smilingly brought me a glass of water.

Mrs. Bono would have curled up in a corner had she witnessed the "Babe" bit. My tablemates and I laughed it off, knowing or hoping matters would soon get back to normal.

The last couple of weeks have been "dry runs" in retailer's talk or "the shake-down cruise" in navy lingo.

December 9, 1985

Christmas season 1985 . . . and once again I feel the heartbeat of the Christmas season. I love the aura that emanates from smiling faces, warm handclasps, and cheery greetings.

There's something about glowing windows, decorated trees, and crisp winter air that stirs within me a longing for home and a return, if only in thought, to a place and time symbolic of love and a *sense of belonging* and well-being.

I long to experience again the warmth of feeling that my home represented. Instead, I'll do my best to bridge my past with the present and make my Christmas here at COTG a pleasant and happy experience. The Christmas seasons fills an emotional need that is buried deep within me.

December 10, 1985

Those of us who danced through the forties to the music of the Big Bands built a "stairway to the stars" last evening, when we listened to *Moonlight Serenade,* a two-hour tribute to Glen Miller. I know I reminisced with pleasure as Tex Benecke conducted the orchestra and Johnny Desmond and Marian Hutton sang. Van Johnson hosted the program of nostalgic music.

December 18, 1985

I haven't made any entries in this journal for several days. I've been mulling over various incidents that occurred here at COTG . . . and hoping, truly hoping, that before I become too old or too complacent to recall or remember the niceties of gracious living, someone will build and staff a *home* that offers services somewhere between those available in a *retirement home* and those services that are necessary in a total care *nursing home.*

Surely there are others who would like the privacy of an attractive room or apartment with available nurse aides and assistance when needed *without* being thought a nuisance or regarded as one of the confused who needs spoonfeeding.

If it weren't for the responsibility of having to hire and maintain my own nursing aide and household staff, I'd rent an apartment and again try my hand at independent living.

I know the above "sputtering" is due to the opening of COTG's new wing and the attendant inconveniences; also, I know that at my age and with my years of work experience, I should be able to take in stride the cavalier, offhand attitude of the in-training new employees, the accidental cutting off of hot water, and the almost unbelievable number of times the fire alarm has been falsely set off or the number of new residents who seemingly can't find their rooms but manage to easily locate mine or, because they are new or inconvenienced by change, argue with one another outside my door or at a nearby table in the dining room.

I'll get over my annoyance and discontent. I always do! Sometimes it takes a bit of doing, but I think I have the remedy this time. Charles Van Doren's new book, *The Joy of Reading*, has just been delivered to me. After reading Van Doren's introduction, I know it won't be too long before I'm lost in its pages; then false fire alarms and careless handling by the new aides won't matter too much.

December 22, 1985

In retrospect, this holiday season hasn't been complete confusion . . . just periodic chaos. But I'm a softie and a sentimentalist, and the temporary inconveniences at COTG will soon be drowned in the rebirth of another Christmas and my cherished memories of happy Christmases of years gone by.

I realize this Christmas can be whatever I want it to be. The key to my contentment will be my ability to bridge the happiness of the past with the reality of today. I know I can bridge that gap by my *acceptance* of the present and my *faith* in the future . . . both of which stem from that birth nearly two thousand years ago, which ushered in a new age of spiritual understanding. It's that understanding that now fills my heart and mind and that I've found so necessary to my living in a nursing home.

Christmas, December 25, 1985

While confusion still reigns at COTG, I just close my door, settle my nose in a book, and let the nursing home world go by. This withdrawal has been happily and pleasantly interrupted today by friends calling and stopping by. My personable young doctor and his fiancée were the last to stop by. Following their departure, I watched and listened to *The Nutcracker* ballet with Mikhail Baryshnikov and later *The Messiah* played by the St. Louis Symphony. Both were on Public Television. Then a bit later back to Van Doren's book. His analysis and depth of understanding of various books and authors convinces me I'm practically a literary illiterate. And here I thought I was a fairly well read person. His book, *The Joy of Reading,* has motivated me to reread many of the books I've read and to start exploring the many books I haven't read.

Today has been again an enjoyable, happy day, and I'm touched deeply by the thoughtfulness and kindness of my friends.

December 29, 1985

Knowing my love of animals, Mrs. Bono gave me a pottery replica of a bassett hound. It's so real-looking with its woebegone yet expectant face and droopy, floppy ears, I placed it on a pillow in front of my TV. Everyone walking into my room at first glance thinks it's a live bassett puppy. I do, too! So much so I'm constantly reminded of the cheerful cherub's comments regarding:

Companions

I wish my dog could talk to me
With thoughts his eyes are big and dark.
How sociable our days would be
If he could speak or I could bark.

I believe "Dawg" and I are both grateful that Mrs. Bono brought us together. We've become good friends! In fact, think I'll call him John, the Bassett as Floyd Reay suggested.

New Year's Eve, December 31, 1985

I had previously arranged with Mrs. Bono for champagne and hors d'oeuvres, and I invited three handicapped residents in wheelchairs to join me in my room for a quiet New Year's Eve gathering. To others on my hall who were confined to their rooms for the evening I sent a glass of champagne and a serving of hors d'oeuvres. From the thanks I received, I know my small soiree kept several oldsters (myself included) from spending a lonely and probably teary evening.

New Year's Day, January 1, 1986

There's a shiny bright new year ahead! I keep thinking my past can be the prologue to this coming year . . . that I can build on my happy experiences and memories and become a living, growing person in today's reality or I can stagnate and turn inward.

As today is Morgan's birthday, I'll opt for living each day to its fullest. I'll enjoy each new day's happenings and start making new memories. That's what he'd want me to do!!

January 5, 1986

The week between Christmas and New Year's this year has been the most pleasurable for me since I came to COTG in December 1979.

Calls, letters, cards, gifts, and visits from friends as well as holiday TV programs opened a floodgate of happy memories for me.

Seeing Dorothy and Floyd Reay yesterday brought back memories of my early years at SBF. The three of us laughed at length as I recalled my introduction to that emporium. The then (it was May 1940) publicity director, J. Walter Goldstein, known affectionately as Scoop, interviewed me. After reviewing my qualifications and background, he offered me the job of writing advertising copy for the store's home division, which headed up to a divisional merchandise manager by the name of Hans Tarrash. Mr. Tarrash was a short, direct, warm-hearted (although you'd never expect that attribute on first encounter), explosive little "Prussian," who, when Mr. Goldstein introduced us, announced in a loud, bombastic voice, "I don't vant a voman. I vant a man for dat job. I don't vant a voman!"

Without going into all the agonizing details, briefly, Mr. Goldstein smoothed my more-amused-than-hurt feelings, I was hired, Mr. Tarrash and I became good friends, and I subsequently spent thirty-three enjoyable years working for old Stix, Baer and Fuller (now Dillards).

Seeing and talking with some of my buyers of years gone by renewed and revitalized those treasured friendships.

As for the holiday programs, listening to the Vienna Philharmonic playing Strauss waltzes and hearing Walter Cronkite talk about and viewing once again the magnificent Lippizaner horses brought out once again the warm memories I have of that tug-at-my-heart city and the *gemütlich* (must remember to ask Kenny Wilde how to spell that word) attitude of the Austrian people.

Last evening, quite by chance, I tuned into a TV program showing scenes of Hong Kong, to me one of the most exotic cities I ever visited. Seeing that beautiful harbor again made me think of the number of times I had crossed it in a Star ferry; and watching the tram crawl upward reminded me of the many times I had journeyed to the Peak. Scenes of Aberdeen, the teeming area housing thousands of boat people, glimpses of sampans plying guests to and from the floating restaurants, and the fountain entrance to the Peninsula Hotel, all rekindled a desire in me to revisit that unique Asian city. Knowing I can't very easily make such a trip now, I settled for the next best thing. I refreshed my memory of Hong Kong history, much of which I still retained . . . and much that I had almost, but not quite, forgotten.

According to my references, Hong Kong's name is derived from "Heung Kong," meaning "Fragrant Harbor," which was the Chinese name for an anchorage at Aberdeen (named for Lord Aberdeen) and so named because ships could take on fresh water from springs nearby.

Kowloon's name means "Nine Dragons" and comes from an incident some eight hundred years ago when boy emperor Ping counted eight hills and remarked that there must be eight dragons, because of the ancient belief that a dragon inhabits every mountain. His prime minister told him there were nine dragons because of another ancient belief that an emperor is a dragon. The name Kowloon has come down through the centuries.

Hong Kong is a British colony consisting of Hong Kong Island, ceded to Britain in 1842, Kowloon Peninsula, ceded from the Chinese in 1860, and the New Territories, leased by Britain in 1898 for ninety-nine years.

Over 99 percent of the population is Chinese, the majority being Cantonese, with that dialect prevailing. English, however, is spoken in all urban areas.

Hong Kong, being within the tropics, has a climate that is in general monsoonal.

The colony's farming is for the most part in the New Territories. Its industry is mostly in Kowloon and the nearby New Territories, its commerce is handled predominantly in the Victoria Central District of Hong Kong, and the residences of the wealthy are in the main on Hong Kong Island.

The Chinese originally smoked opium grown in Western China, but developed a taste for foreign opium when the Portuguese introduced it from India. In the seventeenth century the English, because of their interests in India, built up a sizable trade in it, against the edicts of the Chinese government. The Chinese tried to suppress the illicit opium trade. This was the start of the Opium War, when the English blockaded Canton and occupied the forts there. Through forced negotiations, an agreement was reached. Later, Hong Kong was established as a free port.

On December 8, 1941, the day after Pearl Harbor, the Japanese attacked Hong Kong and effected its surrender.

After the war ended in 1945, the British reestablished control and set up an efficient administration with stable prices and no inflation. This attracted capital from other areas, and it soon became apparent that Hong Kong could no longer rely upon entrêpot trade and emphasis was switched to industry, especially textiles.

Someday I really want to revisit that fascinating city!

January 6, 1986

I had been (still am) enjoying Van Doren's *The Joy of Reading* so much that I impulsively wrote a letter to him to tell him so.

Today's mail brought me one of the most gracious thank you notes I have ever received. Mr. Van Doren is not only an erudite writer and, in my opinion, a giant in literary circles, he's a gracious and kind gentleman. His informal and chatty reply means a great deal to me.

January 10, 1986

And what a beautiful and surprising gift I received today! One dozen roses in an exquisite arrangement came from Julia and Y. D. Chen. The Chens are a charming Chinese couple who were ADG's commissionaires in Hong Kong.

I met and first worked with their office in 1968 and was completely captivated by their knowledge and retail expertise. When I retired from SBF in 1974, they sent me a Chinese ming tree, an exquisite, small decorative tree with blossoms of semiprecious stones and leaves of jade—all set in a jade pot.

Never having accepted any gift of value during my buying years, I was in a quandary as to what to do and how to react to this beautiful gift. I went to Mr. Baer and asked his opinion. Knowing the Chens and their integrity, he told me to accept the gift, that it was one of the loveliest gestures ever made to an SBF buyer.

I'm looking at that beautiful artifact now. I've enjoyed and treasured it for years!

January 17, 1986

I started this journal on December 17, 1984. Today, January 17, 1986, is just one year and one month since I started talking to myself in written form. This journal has not only kept the nursing home walls from caving in on me, it has helped me come to grips with my handicap and has extended my horizons. Today I can be alone and not be lonely. I have learned to savor my memories and friendships as one would taste and appreciate a vintage wine. Too, I now am able to look forward to whatever tomorrows I have left with anticipation and enthusiasm.

I'm continuing to enjoy Van Doren's book. It's good to read, cogitate over, and absorb someone else's thoughts for a change. I think I'm getting a bit bored with conversing with myself. I suspect my journal entries will be sparsely spaced from now on.

January 21, 1986

I always thought of my father as being quite a brilliant man. I knew he was an outstanding college student. As of last Saturday, I learned he had been a very bright little boy also.

My father's grandnephew, of whom he was quite fond, sent me a school report card of my father's dated 1894, when my dad was ten years old.

This nephew of Dad's, James D. Ream, Jr., of Merritt Island, Florida, would be my cousin twice removed (believe that's the way one figures this relationship).

Jim, who since I've known him, has been very interested in the Ream genealogy, is, with his two sons, the last to carry on the Ream name (my maiden name).

But getting back to Dad, this report card of 1894 lists him as being first in his class.

I know my father had to get special permission from the chancellor of the University of Nebraska to enroll there when he was fifteen years old. I know, too, that during his undergraduate years he was a student assistant or instructor teaching both Latin and math.

My paternal grandfather, James D. Ream, Sr., an early settler in the state of Nebraska and a master farmer and one of the leaders of the Nebraska Grange, wanted my father to study or enroll in an agricultural school, but Dad had "wheels" in his head. That caused a rift (later healed) between father and son.

My father paid his college tuition by working and sleeping in a doctor's office. At age nineteen he was state electrician of Nebraska. Later he worked for the Standard Bridge Company (probably no longer in existence), and according to stories that were told me by my mother, he engineeringly changed the course of the Platte River. It seems several attempts had been made to bridge the Platte, at North Platte, I believe. I don't know the problems involved, but for some reason or other, the coffer dams wouldn't hold when the bridge was being built over the water. As the story goes, Dad had the bridge substantially built over dry land, then changed the course of the Platte by damming and sandbagging so that the river flowed under the bridge. As I recall, this was all a matter of record . . . if one could locate the records. Jim Ream might be interested in tracking down the information.

I know, too, my father was thought an excellent engineer, or so Charles Kettering of General Motors said. Mr. Ketterling was instrumental in my father's moving to Dayton, Ohio, in the early 1920s.

I remember my parents with so much love and gratitude. They instilled in me my drive and desire for learning and knowledge. Being an only child, I was treated as an adult and was often brought into my parents' conversations. Whenever a word came up that I didn't understand, I was encouraged to look it up in a huge dictionary that always seemed to be available. I, at that time, thought that book as large as I. My parents would first spell the word. I would locate it in the dictionary, and one or the other of my parents would help me with the definition, if it was beyond me.

A standing joke in the neighborhood where we lived at the time (I was about six years old) concerned my request of a neighbor. I had been given a live baby chick, and I called upon this neighbor to show her my newly acquired little friend and to ask permission to take my chick out on her lawn, explaining that my chick just revelled in good, green grass.

January 25, 1986

There was an article in the *Post-Dispatch* recently titled "Writing Away Stress." The author, Dr. Glen M. Leonard, historian and director of church history and art in Salt Lake City, said: "Diaries can be therapeutic, the way for people to unload their problems and get them off their minds.'

That article caused me to reflect upon my reasons for keeping a diary or journal. Certainly it has been good physical discipline and therapy for me. Too, it unquestionably relieves many of the frustrations that I let become my cross since becoming physically handicapped. I believe, however, I've kept my journal because I like talking to myself. These communiqués to me have helped to keep my attitude and feelings upbeat. As for going back to my journal to relive an event or feeling, I don't do that because it hasn't been necessary. My journal entries have been the reverse. Something I've seen, heard, or read during each new day inspires me to rummage in my memory bank and locate the event, circumstance, or person that the item triggered. I then write about it. In that way, my memory is jogged and my written reminiscences keep those memories fresh and at my fingertips (no pun intended).

Most important, I've found writing in my journal is fun.

January 26, 1986

Eve Wilde sent me an article, "Shanghai: The Vintage Years," by Irene Korbally Kuhn, that has reawakened a long buried wish that I could have enjoyed or at least visited certain cities during their heyday or vintage years. Shanghai is one one of those cities; Budapest is another.

Irene Kuhn, now living in Greenwich Village, was a journalist during the 1920s with the *China Press,* an American-edited, English language newspaper in Shanghai. In her article, Ms. Kuhn brings to life all I've ever read, heard, or thought about as being Shanghaiese—all the qualities of exoticism, color, and excitement she says, however, only existed for a very short time . . . from the start of World War I to the capture of the Japanese part of the city by the Japanese in 1937.

During those years, the city epitomized those qualities. They actually existed then in all their extraordinary variety and complexity.

She says the city was so cosmopolitan that "some thirty nationalities lived and worked there in amiable juxtaposition." The International Settlement was almost a city-state, with its own observed code of law, governed by its own municipal council composed of all resident nationalities; it had its own police force of tall, straightspined, turbaned Sikhs, its own customs, authorities, courts, currency . . . even its own language, "the delightful flexible, easily acquired Pidgin English. . . . But it was the Chinese city, noisy, vast and vibrant with its teeming life and drama surrounding the settlement that really claimed the heart and mind of every Westerner who was fortunate enough to know Shanghai in that brief, suspended time between the wars."

I finished the article feeling the adventurous, enterprising free-spirited life of the city.

Sketching the history of the city, it appears that many years before and under the terms of the Treaty of Nanking (which ended the Opium War in 1842), British merchants were given permission to set up permanent trading establishments and residences in Shanghai as well as in other Chinese cities. The French, Americans, and other nationalities soon followed . . . and the Shanghai International Settlement came into being.

Shanghai, which has existed through wars, revolutions, and decades of isolation, left Irene Kuhn sensing that this life of number one boys, number one cooks, wash and baby amahs, formal entertaining, and all that made up life in that suspended period would never exist again. That, Ms. Kuhn concludes, more than anything else, was what made that brief, bright span "Shanghai's Vintage Years."

January 28, 1986

I have been so annoyed (almost angry) with the carelessness and take-it-or-leave-it attitude of some of the staff members here that I've had to take me over in the corner and give me a good "talking to." I'm calmed down now and have about convinced myself that if it isn't the best of all worlds, at least COTG is really trying to make it a fair facsimile.

Perhaps when Mrs. Bono gets back from her well-deserved month-long vacation, things will get back on smoother running tracks. If not, perhaps by then my throbbing foot (from being carelessly bumped), my insulted derriere (my bottom insulted from being softly [?] dropped), and my injured sensitivities or sensibilities will have all recovered. I've almost talked myself into believing I was the one at fault in each instance. Common sense tells me differently, however.

Oh, well, something nice usually comes along to distract me and take my mind off me. And it did. I have just had delivered to me a complimentary copy of *China Reconstructs.* With my long-time interest in anything Chinese, I'm intrigued with the magazine and am very tempted to subscribe to it, even though I made up my mind a few months ago that I wasn't going to subscribe to another magazine.

It will be interesting to see which wins out . . . my susceptibility or my conservatism.

January 28, 1986, 10:30 A.M. St. Louis time

Eventually everything comes into perspective. Sometimes it takes a heart-rending tragedy . . . an earthquake in Mexico, a terrorist attack in Beirut, Rome, or Vienna, or the just-occurred violent explosion of the *Challenger* to make us all realize how finite we humans are and how trivial our self-centered concerns are.

January 31, 1986

Today was a day of heartfelt national mourning for the *Challenger* astronauts. Across the country, memorial services were held for those seven who dared to expand our knowledge of what we are and how we began and to learn something about that eternity we are probing.

Perhaps we'll never know all the answers. Perhaps we're not supposed to know, but whatever we do glean and learn from these probes into space should take us well beyond the limits of our current perceptions, suppositions, and knowledge. What we learn could very likely shake up many of us and cause us to rethink our opinions and attitudes toward scientific development, religion, personal philosophy, and even death.

I wish I were young enough and able enough to qualify for the space program. I'd jump at the chance to even be considered. All of which makes me realize that I've come to terms with my handicap, that I've accepted my advancing years, but growing old *beyond my usefulness* is difficult for me to rationalize.

February 2, 1986

Yesterday at luncheon, two elderly gentlemen at the next table were having a lively discussion about the pleasures of fishing. The topic quickly moved from mud cats in the Mississippi to scavenger fish in general. One gentleman remarked that carp were "good eating" if properly prepared and cooked. The other gentleman was dubious. I was reminded of a recipe I once heard about:

1. Select a clean, smooth board (preferably oak), about three-quarters of an inch thick.
2. Grease one side of the board well with either butter or cooking oil.
3. Salt and pepper oiled side of board.

4. Place thoroughly cleaned and seasoned carp on board.
5. Arrange three strips of bacon across fish.
6. Bake in 350 degree oven for one hour.
7. Remove from oven, discard fish, and eat board.

February 3, 1986

I've been chuckling over a Xeroxed work study report mailed to me by Joan Shaw, music therapist at COTG. I don't know who wrote it. The only identification on the report says: "Circulated anonymously among employees of the British Ministry of Transport." A footnote on the report concludes: "From the Bulletin of American Association of University Professors, Autumn 1955."

The Report of a Work Study Engineer after a Visit to a Symphony Concert at the Royal Festival Hall in London.

For considerable periods the four oboe players had nothing to do. The number should be reduced and the work spread more evenly over the whole of the concert, thus eliminating peaks of activity.

All the twelve violins were playing identical notes; this seems unnecessary duplication. The staff of this section should be drastically cut. If a larger volume of sound is required, it could be obtained by means of electronic apparatus.

Much effort was absorbed in the playing of demi-semi-quavers; this seems to be an unnecessary refinement. It is recommended that all notes should be rounded up to the nearest semi-quaver. If this were done, it would be possible to use trainees and lower-grade operatives more extensively.

There seems to be too much repetition of some musical passages. Scores should be drastically pruned. No useful purpose is served by repeating on the horns a passage which has already been handled by the strings. It is estimated that if the redundant passages were eliminated, the whole concert time of 2 hours could be reduced to 20 minutes and there would be no need for an intermission.

The conductor agrees generally with these recommendations, but expresses the opinion that there might be some falling off in box-office receipts. In that unlikely event, it should be possible to close sections of the auditorium entirely, with a consequential saving of overhead expenses, lighting, attendants, etc. If the worst came to the worst, the whole thing could be abandoned and the public could go to the Albert Hall instead.

Following the principle that "there is always a better method," it is felt that further review might still yield additional benefits. For example, it is considered that there is still wide scope for application of the Questioning Attitude to many of the methods of operation, as they are in many cases traditional and have not been changed for many centuries.

In the circumstances it is remarkable that Methods Engineering principles have been adhered to as well as they have. For example, it was noted that the pianist was not only carrying out most of his work by two-handed operation, but was also using both feet for pedal operations. Nevertheless, there were excessive reaches for some notes on the piano and it is probable that re-design of the keyboard to bring all notes within the normal working area would be of advantage to this operator. In many cases the operators were using one hand for holding the instrument whereas the use of a fixture would have rendered the idle hand available for other work.

It was noted that excessive effort was being used occasionally by the players of wind instruments, whereas one air compressor could supply adequate air for all instruments under more accurately controlled conditions.

Obsolescence of equipment is another matter into which it is suggested further investigation could be made, as it was reputed in the program that the leading violinist's instrument was already several hundred years old. If normal depreciation schedules had been applied the value of this instrument should have been reduced to zero and it is probable that purchase of more modern equipment could have been considered.

February 15, 1986

It had to be because of the day, Valentine's Day. I was on a sentimental journey all day yesterday. It started in the morning when Mrs. Bono gave each resident a corsage or boutonniere. Then like a silly schoolgirl I started rereading the messages on the valentines I'd received.

I finished off the evening by sniffling through a rerun of Eric Segal's tender but soggy *Love Story*. At 2: 00 A.M. I decided it was time I acted my age and went to sleep. Whispering, "Good night, Morgan," I snuggled under the covers.

February 18, 1986

Because I liked Ms. Kuhn's article on Shanghai, I wrote a note to her telling her so. Today I received a gracious thank you note enclosing a reprint of two other articles she had written and thought I might enjoy. I could and did relate to both articles.

One told about her love of travel and some of her interesting experiences. The other, titled "Friends for All Seasons," particularly struck a responsive chord in me. She likened her friends to the seasons of the year:

There were those who like springtime were bubbly and effervescent. Those are the young people in the springtime of their lives. They share their hopes and dreams and give us an opportunity to relive our own young years when we were full of promise and adventure.

Then there are her summer friends "men and women I have known for many years." She felt those friendships were "as full of the richness and bounty of life as is the summertime." Those, I believe, are the ones that have come to full flowering.

The autumn friends Ms. Kuhn says are her wonderful long-time cronies. They, she feels, are as colorful as the foliage of fall. Winter friendships are her friends who are "old in years but not in spirit." They are still accomplishing and have a zest for living.

I've never compared my friends and friendships to the seasons, but how apt that comparison is when you think about it.

February 19, 1986

I've been nursing viral pleurisy for several days, and I'm so cranky and irritable I can't even stand myself. But to build up my self-image a bit . . . I know I do so much for myself I often don't get the assistance I really need. That just happened to me, and I didn't take the neglect with the grace I would have liked to have shown.

February 21, 1986

This A.M. the director of activities, Delores Silies, took three of us to an open rehearsal of the St. Louis Symphony. Raymond Leppard conducted.

I particularly liked the Eroica, Beethoven's Third in E flat major. Much as I enjoyed the music, I was "bushed" by the time we arrived back at COTG at 2: 00 P.M.

February 25, 1986

I'm one of the millions of ordinary people who is vitally interested in what is going on in this screwed up world of ours. As a result of

this interest, I have become a newscast and panel discussion addict.
Whether it's the MacNeil-Lehrer program, William Buckley's "Firing
Line," David Brinkley, or just plain Joe Blow, I enjoy listening to and
thinking about the divergent opinions expressed.

There's only one discussion group, the McLaughlin Group, I find
so annoying I seldom listen to them (or it) anymore.

Why intelligent men can't discuss issues without rudely inter-
rupting one another or shouting an opposing opinion I'll never know.

To me, the McLaughlin Group sounds more like a female kaf-
feeklatsch or a roomful of noisy, bickering siblings than a panel of
serious-minded men interested in world happenings.

March 4, 1986

"Yes," I answered Mickie, "there are times I'd like to throw
things—or sit in the middle of the floor and pound my heels on the
floor (if I only could) or just scream.

"But what good would that do? It won't bring Morgan back and
the life I once knew. I have sense enough to know I must make a
new life for myself with what I have to work with *now.*"

Dreams, memories, music, friendships, books, goals, and as-
pirations are some of the tools I use to create many pleasant hours.
Pleasant and enjoyable hours can be made into a happy day, I've
found. And that isn't too difficult to do. I just keep reminding myself
that I don't think God is through with me yet . . . and I keep plodding
along.

March 9, 1986

As I wheeled myself back from the dining room this noon, I
paused for a few minutes to observe the oldsters gathered around the
central nurses' desk. Most were in wheelchairs. Some were seated
in chairs against the wall of the skylight rotunda under which the
nurses' desk is located. Others were ambling aimlessly around.

I couldn't help thinking, *How hauntingly sad . . . and how
hauntingly beautiful.*

Here was embodied years of accomplishment, years of priceless,
really valuable experience. Here was a cross-section of life with its
accumulation of laughter, tears, joy, and heartbreak . . . an accumulation of successes and failures.

When I returned to my room, I whispered, "Please, dear God,
help me *not* to vegetate. Help me to remain aware of what is going

on in the world. Help me to contribute if I can, and please let me know when I can't. Please, dear God, *don't* let me become a care or burden to anyone."

I don't think my insufferable pride could take that.

March 25, 1986

I've done little or no writing for a couple of weeks—for several reasons:

1. My room looks as though a bomb had hit it! Earlier I had decided I either had to move or clean house. I couldn't believe I had accumulated so much "stuff" since coming to COTG, but I have. I've discovered, too, that reorganizing closets, chest drawers, and my desk (even with assistance) is a long, tiring process when directed from a wheelchair. Do I throw that away? Should I keep this? If so, where do I put it?
2. The hanging of new wallpaper, changing light fixtures, and the rearranging of my furniture and rugs has only added to the confusion. I'm looking forward to next week, when I hope my room will have taken on some semblance of a quiet, restful home.

Easter Sunday, March 30, 1986

I believe we all go through, in some small way or other, our crucifixions and resurrections. I believe most of us go through these temporary deaths and rebirths many times during our life. These transformations may relate or appertain to our spiritual outlook, our emotional responses, our physical well-being . . . or our attitudes in general.

My most recent experience started several days ago. It continued through Good Friday, March 28, and up to today, Easter Sunday, March 30. Because of my physical inability to do the many things I wanted to do—take steps by myself, reach a book I wanted, even sit or lie down without assistance—I let my frustrations alter my attitude from upbeat to one of dejection. I began thinking how futile it was to try to create a few pleasant hours that I could make into a happy day. Up to that point, I hadn't created a single happy hour that day. It was then a fellow resident stopped by to see me. Her attitude was so much more depressed than mine that before I knew it, I was comforting her. Later on in the day, that same resident invited me to her room and we listened to a taped reading of Dr. Buscaglia's "Bus 9 to Paradise." In the evening I watched and listened to uplifting words and music, my faith in me and life was restored. Before that I had about decided I was being silly to think God isn't through with me yet.

Today, Easter Sunday, I am again convinced that I can be as happy as I want to be or I can be as miserable as I *let* myself be. And I'm too old to start being miserable again!

March 31, 1986

I'm looking at a framed Japanese batik hanging above my desk. I bought it in Kyoto and I'm reminded once again of that beautiful ancient city. Not only is Kyoto the heart of Japanese Buddhism and the site of hundreds of Shinto shrines, it is also the center of Japan's culture and art.

For over a thousand years, Kyoto was the seat of the imperial government. It was called Heian Kyo . . . meaning City of Peace and Tranquillity. Perhaps that name was prophetic, as it came through World War II unscathed.

While no longer the seat of government, Kyoto still wears an aura of imperialism and detached elegance.

I remember so well the Kiyomizu Temple and the Heian Shrine, the Golden and Silver Pavilions, the Silk Museum, and the pampered carp in the lovely garden lake back of the museum. The carp practically jumped from the water to grab bread sticks from my hand.

And I'll never forget the rainy Sunday Eiko and Toshio Sannaka took me sightseeing. For me it was a beautiful day because of their friendly interest and kindness. And I'm certain there are many Americans who will always remember courtly, gracious Mr. T. Shimo, lovingly called Jimmy San. Then he was owner or director of Kyo Trading Company. I have no idea how old Mr. Shimo was. I know he was far from young. He had lived in the United States for some time, and he laughingly told me how he had acquired a taste for sauerkraut. He and Mrs. Shimo while over here had hired a German cook, and it wasn't long before Mr. Shimo found himself preferring sauerkraut to sushi.

To top off my day of reminiscing about Japan, its beauty, and my Japanese friends, in the evening I watched a rerun of *Sayonara*. No wonder I went to sleep thinking of geishas, beautiful gardens, crazy cab drivers, and my frequent plea to them of "Yukuro dozo" (Easy, please).

April 1, 1986

Because my thinking is very fuzzy about the naming of April Fool's Day, I think I'll call the public library and get my facts straight. Somehow I keep thinking the changing to the Gregorian calendar had something to do with it, but just how, why, or when I don't recall.

I called the library and learned: In 1564 France changed the date of New Year's from April 1 to January 1. Those persons who continued to adhere to the April first date were referred to as "April fools." The English took up the expression, and that's how it spread and became fixed.

April 14, 1986

Not too long ago I told Ken Wilde about the gracious thank you letter I'd received from Charles Van Doren. I had previously written to Mr. Van Doren telling him how much I was enjoying his new book, *The Joy of Reading*. Ken, knowing my admiration for Ronald Reagan, said he wondered if President Reagan would answer my letter if I wrote to him. I wondered, too, so I wrote a brief letter to him.

I told him that although for physical reasons it was necessary for me to live in a nursing home, I still tried to keep abreast of what was going on in the world and that I was very happy I had voted for him in '80 and '84 and would do so again if it were possible for him to seek another term.

Today's mail just brought me a personal letter from President Reagan. Following is his letter. (Like some star-struck teenager, I'm thinking of having his letter framed.)

THE WHITE HOUSE
Washington
April 11, 1986

Dear Mrs. Schwind:

You were very kind to send along your thoughtful greetings and generous words. I was sorry to learn of your health problems, but it's clear you have a strong and caring spirit that sees you through life's challenges and then some.

May I return your kindness and assure you that Nancy and I will cherish your friendship and keep you in our thoughts and prayers.

God bless you.

Sincerely,
Ronald Reagan

April 15, 1986

It's the last day for filing '85 tax returns. Mercantile filed mine a month ago. Annoyed by the tax I had to pay? No. I'm grateful my income was sufficient to be taxable.

Last evening, 4/14, at 7:00 P.M. E.S.T. the U.S. fired upon Libyan installations.

April 18, 1986

The *verbal* flack over the Libyan raid continues to land around us. Some of this flack is good—much is not so good. I have a feeling, however, that when the dust settles down, our allies will start taking a stronger stand against Libya and terrorism in general. Too, I think the Soviets are too smart to scuttle the hoped-for summit meeting.

Everyone regrets that there were some civilian victims as a result of our bombing.

April 21, 1986

Last evening I watched the Television Academy induct seven outstanding personalities into its Hall of Fame. I was particularly interested because Frank Stanton, a former CBS president, was one of the seven inducted.

I knew Frank 'way back when in high school in Dayton, Ohio. When I was a freshman at Stivers High, Frank was a junior at Steele High School. Ruth Stevenson, whom he later married, was a schoolmate of mine at Stivers High. She was a junior. I was a lowly freshman; however, neither Ruth nor Frank ever treated me as such.

Many years after I married I asked a favor of Frank, which he promptly granted. When Robert Stephan of the *Cleveland Plain Dealer* died (Bob was Morgan's brother-in-law), Arthur Godfrey paid Bob a beautiful tribute on his radio show. Knowing how much Morgan and his sister cared, I wrote Frank asking if it were possible for

170

me to obtain a transcript of Godfrey's words. Frank immediately sent me a record containing all of Godfrey's comments. Morgan and his sister, as well as I, were deeply touched by Frank's kindness.

April 29, 1986

The article "Earthquake in Mexico" in the May issue of *National Geographic* makes me wonder if such tragedies, earthquakes, volcanic eruptions, floods, famines, et cetera, aren't nature's way of cautioning man about his follies: the fast track the world is taking toward overpopulation, man's misuse of nature's bounties, and his often total disregard of nature's plan of balance.

Whether stupid or erudite, such questions give me something to mull over.

April 29, later

Listening to all the various newscasts today about the Russian nuclear "mishap" in the Ukraine makes me think perhaps man's manipulation of nature (splitting the atom, et cetera) is another warning of man's carelessness in handling nature's largess.

April 29, evening

The New York Philharmonic's concert this evening soon dispelled all my thoughts of nuclear meltdowns and earthquakes. Zubin Mehta conducted. Montserat Caballe, soprano, and Itzhak Perlman and Isaac Stern, violinists, were the guests artists. It was truly a gala concert!

Wouldn't it be wonderful if music were really the world's common denominator . . . instead of anxiety, fear, and politics?

May 4, 1986

Yesterday was Derby Day. I kept wishing I could be in Louisville for the 112th running of the Kentucky Derby. Since I couldn't be there, I did the next best thing. I picked a horse and bet with Nell DeF——, who enjoys the Derby as much as I.

We didn't attend a single Derby breakfast, dinner, or dance or have even one mint julep, but we had a fun time.

I lost! Nell was much smarter than I. She chose and bet on the jockey. I was scientific and bet on the name that intrigued me. "Fobby Forbes" still tickles my fancy. I think he's still running!

Even so, I must mail a one-dollar bill to Nell. Never let it be said I don't pay my gambling debts.

May 7, 1986

One of the residents said she had been watching TV shots of the Breakers, the famous Cornelius Vanderbilt "cottage" overlooking the Atlantic at Newport. I remember seeing it from Sturgis Rice's yacht. That was the closest I ever came to the Breakers, but thinking about Newport, Vanderbilt, Astor, et cetera, reminded me of the term "four hundred" and the bit of free verse (quite free, I must admit) that I wrote when I was society editor of the *Dayton Journal-Herald* and wrote under the byline of Wanda Ream.

I rummaged through my file and found it. It was written, I believe, in 1937. Now I'm wondering how many of the families mentioned are still there. It has been so many years since I've been back to Dayton!

Written by Wanda Ream (Schwind) in 1937. At the time she was Society Editor of the Dayton Journal-Herald *and wrote a column called "Over the Teacups" under the byline Wanda Ream.*

There are towns that show no pavements on their streets—
No shaded lawns or parks or architectural treats
Of grandeur to display. But try to find
A city or a village or a town of any kind
That doesn't flaunt a special set of its society—
A "gayer few" who've grown into an aristocracy.
You have heard the words "four hundred" tossed about
More freely than election, Mrs. Simpson or the drought—
These words that have been frequently applied
To groups whose actual numbers would divide
The term in half, and then again to signify
A set whose membership would doubly multiply
The appellation. What's the meaning of it all?
Who invented the barometer of social rise and fall?
The origin is buried in a maze of famous names
In an adolescent era when the most ambitious dames

Fought deadly battles on the famous fields of Newport—
And the crisis of the war was the deafening report
Heard 'round the social world, the real disaster—
The social cannon fired in '82 by Mrs. William Astor
When she arbitrarily issued the command
To cut her guest list to include a tiny band
Of just "four hundred" persons—not one more
And the rest were left forlornly on the shore
Of social failure. So was born the practice of exclusion,
The traditional "four hundred"—our numerical confusion.

And so each town's "four hundred" has survived
Since the bustle days from which it has derived
Its real significance. In Dayton it may be
A group that numbers more than the allotted coterie—
But it's still the old "four hundred," and we're proud
Of the lengthy list that represents the crowd
Of first-edition families—names that grew
In healthy soil when entertaining was a new
Diversion in a straggling, awkward town—
Names of men who started things and handed down
To us our heritage. And names of recent birth,
Whose possessors have been quick to prove their worth
By contributing to Dayton's social health,
Her industrial existence or her economic wealth.
Names that glitter in the headlines of the city's social notes
But are capable of grinning and throwing off their coats
And working toward a common goal of man's prosperity—
These are name that are important in an aristocracy.

In the roster of our city, we see with just a glance
The Pattersons, the Estabrooks, the Simonds and the Grants;
The Gardners and the Stanleys, the Reynolds and the Slacks,
The Whittakers, the Ketterings, the Kittredges and Flacks;
The Gebharts and the Fowlers, and the Harrisons and Bunns,
The Biechlers and the Thackers, Cleggs and Robinsons—
The list goes on and on, and we are properly impressed
With the crowded population in the land of Dayton's best.
We might say we'd mention all if we weren't limited by time—
But that's a lie—the truth is that we're running out of rhyme.

May 8, 1986

I've never read any of Dr. Wayne Dyer's books, but from an article I read about him today, I like the way he thinks. Dr. Dyer, a well-known proponent of mental health, is quoted as saying that we are the sum total of the choices we've made in our lives. Every emotion we experience in our lives is a choice! Guilt, worry, blame, and depression are irresponsible choices that take up a great deal of time and life energy that keep us from living at the highest level we can achieve.

Dr. Dyer further states that the highest form of sanity is appreciating and savoring each moment. He continues: ". . . we will always be frustrated if we are living any other moment but the present."

I believe so much in living each day to its fullest that I couldn't help but agree. How else could we make happy memories for tomorrow?

May 10, 1986

Today I am seventy-eight years old! I have received so many reminders of how rich I am friendship-wise: books, flowers, candy, cards, phone calls, and friends who took time to visit me. I am deeply touched and keep thinking how blessed I am! I hope if I ever forget that, someone will bat me soundly over the head.

Last evening COTG held its mother-daughter banquet. Those of us having no daughters invited a guest. I chose Rosemary Stratmeyer, a lovely young woman who lost her mother just three months ago. She was such a devoted daughter and misses her mother so much I thought she might like to be my adopted daughter for an evening. Apparently she did, as she thanked me many times during the evening.

The dinner was delicious and the entertainment was especially good. Each resident was given a lovely long-stemmed rose when she entered the dining room.

Each table for four had a flower arrangement. The place cards were hand-painted and charming. Each guest was given an attractive engraved glass coffee mug. I am using mine as a pencil cup for my desk—thus I am frequently reminded of a very pleasant evening.

The dinner menu was as follows:

Tossed salad
Cheese platter
Relish platter
Chicken Waterloo
Wild rice
Green beans
Croissant rolls
Chocolate cup with strawberries
Hawaiian cooler
Coffee—tea

The award-winning Kirkwood chapter of the Sweet Adelines entertained with a program of nostalgic songs dating back to the twenties and World War I.

May 13, 1986

About ten of us were taken to hear Canadian Brass last evening at Powell Symphony Hall. I loved every minute of the concert! I don't think I've ever heard better musicianship.

Five men with two trumpets and one each with French horn, trombone and tuba played everything from Bach, Vivaldi, Handel, Purcell, and Pagannini to Dixieland—and all done with a touch of humor and whimsy.

Today eight of us (COTG residents) visited the museum of the Missouri Historical Society. It had been years since I had been in the Jefferson Memorial, where the museum is housed, and I had forgotten what wonderful treasures the museum contained.

I strolled (wheelchaired) through the Portrait Gallery and the Veiled Prophet Gallery and spent a long time looking at the pictorial and documentary exhibition showing Jewish life in America. This was a new and informative display illustrating the development and contribution of Jews in America from their arrival in New Amsterdam in 1654 to the present. The display consisted of vivid photographic reproductions of prints, paintings, and artifacts from noted institutions across the country.

There were, however, three other exhibits that fascinated me even more, probably because each personally touched a period or time in my life. The Lindbergh exhibit brought back memories of my newspaper days with the *Dayton Journal-Herald.* I had just gone to the city desk, for some reason or other, when word came over the wire that the Lindbergh baby had been kidnapped. Everyone in the room was stunned. I remember that I cried.

Seeing the bronze busts of the Stix, Baer and Fuller founders, Julius Baer, Sigmund Baer, Charles Stix, and Aaron Fuller, couldn't help but recall my working days (thirty-three years) with that fine old family firm, known as Stix, Baer and Fuller.

When SBF was sold to the Dillards department store chain, "Cubby" (Julius A. Baer II) donated the busts and a bronze water fountain (a gift from SBF employees to Arthur Baer (Cubby's father) to the Missouri Historical Society. All pieces are on prominent display in the museum.

The third display that brought back memories was that of the reconstructed wheelhouse of the *Golden Eagle.* Shortly after Morgan and I came to St. Louis in 1940, we took a three-day excursion on the *Golden Eagle,* the last packet boat on the Mississippi. Although I've been on ocean liners and cruise ships since, none left a deeper impression than that old sternwheeler.

Over the years, there were many moonlit nights that I remember, but I don't think any held more heartfelt love and romance than those moonlit evenings when Morgan and I held hands and watched the silvered shimmering waters of the Mississippi slip by. In the near distance was the muffled splash of the big sternwheel.

I know now that dreams were made on nights like that.

May 17, 1986

I try to learn something new every day. Today I learned a lot!

On May 3, 1986, the Venice Simplon-Orient Express inaugurated service to Istanbul, augmenting its thirty-two-hour sentimental journey from London to Venice. (Pre–World War II, the run was Paris to Istanbul.)

During the years following World War II and my retirement in 1974, I rode the OE many times. Then, though slightly tarnished, she was still the Grande Dame of railroads, plying her way from Paris to Venice and still reflecting much of her former grandeur.

According to an article I just read, an American entrepreneur, James B. Sherwood, rescued the aging lady and, after much "haggling at auctions and spending 5 years on costly repairs," she was returned to the rails in 1983.

Last fall a dramatic Alpine route, passing through Swiss valleys and mountains and picturesque Austrian villages and crossing the Brenner Pass, was added to the regular Italian run. This became so successful it has become a permanent route to Venice, with several ski stops along the way at Zurich, Chur, et cetera, in Switzerland and Innsbruck and St. Anton in Austria.

Today, according to the article, one can entrain at London's bustling Victoria Station, ride to the coast, and board the Channel ferry via red carpeted pathways. Three hours later at Boulogne "One peers to see *THE* train, the *REAL* Orient Express," now one half-mile of gleaming blue and gold cars.

Each car differs in age, origin, and interior theme. Some feature popular motifs, delicate flowers, dancing nymphs, et cetera. Others are enhanced with black lacquer, mother-of-pearl inlay, or Lalique glass. All are outfitted with heavy pewter and polished brass.

It seems everything is beautifully orchestrated and a journey on the Venice Simplon-Orient Express is an elegant example of once-upon-a-time travel, with gourmet food, fresh flowers, and "tinkling piano music." All the trappings of yesteryear are "stunningly re-stored."

While I'd like very much to enjoy this newly restored plush train, I'm glad I had the opportunity to know it when it was still the *real* Orient Express.

May 23, 1986

Joan Shaw, COTG's charming music therapist, often shares bits of philosophy, humor, or whimsy with me. Today she brought me the following reprint of William Childress's column:

Ozark Symphony Croaks Along

It is frustrating to be close to a great attraction but unable to market it properly.

One evening, as I listened to the careful tuning of about 1,000 frogs, I reflected that if I had just half as many people as the St. Louis Symphony, I could make the McDonald County Frog Symphony world-famous, too.

You haven't heard of the McDonald County Frog Symphony? Well, have you heard of the celebrated Jumping Frog of Calaveras County, which Mark Twain reported on some years ago?

We are a natural offshoot of that.

Urban symphonies have a saturation of public-relations folks to keep budgets vibrant and shows going on, but we're the victims of envy. That's my explanation, and I stick to it. The folks who are keen to keep Mark Twain's Frog report alive don't want any competition.

There is no legitimate excuse for keeping McDonald County frogs off the national scene. In the matter of symphonic excellence, they have no match. Let me give you a sampling of a program our frogs put on after a recent rain.

First came the spring peepers, tiny, grating fifes whose music is carried through the velvet dusk for fully half a mile. Acoustics? Why, these boys never heard of such. They need no artificial aids, as human symphonies do.

These little frogs are small, and that is a necessary safety margin. If they were as big as their voices, they could crush houses.

Another big difference between frog music and symphony is that the frogs require much less time to tune up.

They appear to have done the ordinary stuff and are ready at once to serenade. Now I know that music lovers everywhere will leap to their feet and cry, "But half of the tuning up is just for show!"

I don't care. In my opinion, the frogs carry it.

Spurred by the spring peepers, the cricket frogs start clicking. Without a conductor—without a conductor!—they establish and maintain a marvelous rhythm. Cricket frogs put a lot of energy into every performance—and I have known oboe players who could learn from them.

Now the medley is reinforced by chorus frogs—their actual name and job description. Finally, with majestic reluctance, the mighty bullfrogs come in like runaway tubas.

It is the signal for an explosion of decibels like nothing you've heard, so fiercely bright and tymphanic the night seems to sparkle with sound. It is frog symphony at its finest.

You may say what you please, but the McDonald County Frog Symphony can strut its stuff just as ably as the St. Louis Symphony and no PR is necessary to whet the public's appetite, either.

And just because we are rustics, do not imagine that we are ignorant of dress codes.

All our frogs wear tuxedos. They wear them year-round, and each one is form-fitting. What's more, they're not all the same.

I'd like to see an urban symphony top that.

While reading that delightful article by Childress, I was transported back to Echo Valley, our beloved farm in the foothills of the Ozarks. Morgan and I frequently said that we hung our hats at our home in St. Louis, but we *lived* at Echo Valley.

We had a croaking symphony, too, which was at its best after a summer rain. Often of an evening following the frogs' serenade, we were lulled to sleep by the whippoorwill chorus.

I'll admit rustic music like this takes a bit of getting "used to," but once one does, no symphony or chorus plays sweeter music or leaves one with happier memories.

May 24, 1986

While rummaging through my desk this morning, I ran across my 1979 Day Book, which I had sparsely annotated. Glancing through it and recalling some of the events I have deliberately tried to forget, I wonder now how I managed to come through that year as well as I did.

The year had started off with a sleet storm that continued off and on, with snow and icy weather alternating through most of January or at least up to and through January 17, when a stroke caught up with me.

Up to that point in January, I had been pretty much confined to my home, where I was doing my best to overcome my loneliness and the void left by Morgan's absence.

On January 17, 1979, I had gone outside to see if the driveway needed to be snow-plowed again. As I started to walk across the lawn, I felt a numbing sensation in my left foot and hand. I stumbled back to the house, where I fell on my way to the phone. I crawled to a small chair by the telephone and managed to get into the chair. I called Dr. Norman Drey, who told me to stay where I was, that he'd be at my home in minutes. He was! Following my directions in locating robe and slippers, he packed an overnight bag for me, and within a very short time I was in an ambulance and on my way to the hospital.

Between January 17, 1979, and July 31, 1979, when I returned home for good, I hoped, I spent seventy-two days at Jewish Hospital and twenty-seven days at a nearby nursing home (Bernard West).

During those six months, spent mostly on my back or in a wheel-chair, I arranged for household and nursing help and kept the farm going by phone. I sold Echo Valley and signed the final papers on August 3, 1979.

It was during this period that my doctor, Norman Drey, my CPA, Jim Germanese, and my attorney, Bob Meyer, met at my home to urge me to go to a nursing home. I was told I had to get out from under all responsibility. I wasn't too receptive, but I listened, as reliable help was getting increasingly difficult to find.

No one could have had more supportive friends than I had. They researched nursing homes for me, took me to see several, and visited me often. I was surprised by the action of only one. Early on March 6, 1979, according to my Day Book entry, she called to say she'd come to my home and take care of me *if* I'd designate her as my legal guardian and turn over all my financial affairs to her. My answer was no.

I arranged for a young couple, Mr. and Mrs. Guilermo Gomez, to live in my home with me. With their help and that of nurse aides and therapists, I managed quite well. By October, with the help of my attorney and CPA, I had set up a trust fund, narrowed my choice of nursing homes down to two (Marie de Ville and Clayton-on-the-Green), disposed of most of my possessions, and found good homes for my four dogs. The latter broke my heart because aside from loving them for themselves (and they me), they were my last link with Morgan.

Calyton-on-the-Green had an opening first and I moved into that nursing home on December 4, 1979.

As of today, May 26, 1986, I've been at COTG six years, five months, and twenty-two days.

May 28, 1986

One of Bill Cosby's comments made on a talk show recently gave me the answer I've been seeking for quite some time.

I've never had my ears pierced. When asked "Why not?" by women who usually have pierced ears, I answer, "I just never wanted to have it done," thinking the matter would end there. It seldom does, as the questioner often starts in telling me all the advantages of having pierced ears. It's then I'd like to say to the pierced-ear female, "I don't see much difference between piercing my ears and piercing my nose for a nose ring."

I've never made that reply. Instead I just stand there with a silly smile on my face, because I really don't have a good reason. Now I'll borrow from Cosby and say, "I've always been afraid my ears would rot off if I had them pierced."

May 31, 1986

And still another new aide on the evening shift! Hoping to make it easier for her in transferring me, I went into my usual little speech to new aides. I explained that my left side was paralyzed but that I had considerable strength on my right side and that if she'd help me keep my weight and balance on that side, I could pivot on my right foot and all she needed to do was guide me in the transfer.

She smiled and asked, "Did you have a stroke?"

I answered, "Yes."

She then asked, "Did it affect your brain?"

I was slightly nonplussed but replied, "I don't think so."

"That's funny," she said. "My uncle had a stroke and he was nuts afterward."

June 1, 1986

Shades of Edna Ferber's classic novel and the stage play *Showboat*.

Today eighteen residents and four staff members in two COTG vans were taken to the waterfront where we boarded the *Golden Rod*, the last authentic Mississippi River showboat still in regular year-round operation.

After a delicious luncheon in the Captain's Dining Room, we adjourned to the boat's theater, where we were entertained by a musical production, *Josephine's Paris,* which depicted highlights and songs in the theatrical career of Josephine Baker.

Josephine Baker, as most of us knew, was the talented black girl who rose to international fame by *ignoring* the obstacles in her rise to the top from a St. Louis ghetto. She counted kings, queens, and presidents among her friends. It was Princess Grace of Monaco who financed her comeback appearance two days before her death in April 1975. I was fortunate to have seen her once in Paris many years ago.

But more about the *Golden Rod.* According to my references, it was built in September 1909 at a cost of seventy-five thousand. The restoration cost $350,000.

She is the largest showboat ever built. Her original dimensions were two hundred feet long by thirty-five feet wide. The original theater capacity was fourteen hundred persons, making her the largest floating theater in the world. In 1968 the U.S. Department of the Interior designated the *Golden Rod* as a Registered National Historic Landmark.

June 5, 1986

Engineering feats intrigue me, probably because both my father and husband were engineers and I always thought that each could accomplish almost any difficult task.

I read recently that in a year the English Channel tunnel will be well on its way. That, I understand, will be the largest civil engineering project of the twentieth century.

The go-ahead for the construction of the twin thirty-one-mile-long railroad tunnels—131 feet beneath the seabed of the English Channel—was received earlier this year. On January 20, 1986, in Lille, France, French president Mitterand and British prime minister Thatcher announced approval of the winning tunnel design. The following month in Britain's Canterbury Cathedral, a treaty permitting the project to begin was signed. Mr. Mitterand, I'm told, reminded the audience that Napoleon had dreamed of a tunnel two centuries ago. Although the tunnels are financed by private capital, approval of both governments was required.

The tunnels are to be used by conventional freight and passenger trains, as well as special rail shuttle cars that will carry autos and other vehicles, portal to portal.

I wonder, does this mean Britain sees itself and its future tied more to the continent, especially to the expanding economic power of the Common Market? I wonder.

According to a Reuters dispatch, not everyone in Britain is pleased with the "Chunnel Decision." According to Reuters: "For a nation that once believed it was set apart from Continental Europe by some divine right, the impact of a 'fixed link' is profound."

British history has been uniquely shaped by the "Channel Moat." Apparently it was Britain's fear of losing its defensive wall that sealed the fate of the first attempt to bore a rail tunnel in 1883. An expert in railways at that period wrote: "There is the feeling in many breasts that the stormy bulwark God has placed around the Coast should not be undermined." The feeling still persists. Recently a reader wrote to a British newspaper: "If God had meant there to be a 'fixed link' he would have provided a causeway." Nonetheless, barring unforeseen circumstances, the channel tunnel should be in operation by 1993.

After that, will there be a new, uncertain chapter in British history? I can't help but wonder.

June 8, 1986

I keep thinking about the delightful day I had last Wednesday (June 4, 1986) at Highcroft Ridge School. Continuing the program sponsored by the school and COTG, about eight of us visited Highcroft again this year.

We toured the school, participated in games with the children, and were entertained at a delicious fried chicken luncheon with music and songs by the youngsters.

How proud Dr. Richard Overfelt (school principal) must be of his students and the teaching staff! And how proud the parents should be that their children have the opportunity to attend a school like Highcroft.

An atmosphere of creativity and resourcefulness permeates the classrooms. That, coupled with the obvious fact that learning basics is emphasized, gives me the feeling that Highcroft is attaining those almost forgotten standards of learning and growing so desired by parents and educators.

June 14, 1986

I've just finished reading Lewis H. Lapham's essay "Imperial Masquerade," his Notebook contribution in the July issue of *Harper's Magazine*.

I've always enjoyed and admired his writing. Whether I agreed with him or not, I thought his comments fair, analytical, frequently witty, but basically kind. "Imperial Masquerade," I thought was beneath him and hardly journalistic statesmanship.

I carefully reread the article to be certain I wasn't being equally smug in my appraisal of his attitude. I've decided my reaction is just as narrow, as I've ended up thinking, *Now those are the words of a young man (he's probably middle-aged) trying to be "cute" in an effort to attract the attention of the literati.*

I still believe, however, that he is wise enough and empathetic enough to puncture the complacency of the "American Plutocracy" without resorting to ridicule and sarcasm.

June 21, 1986

It was pleasantly warm and the soft summer breeze whispering across the open air theater made last Tuesday evening a perfect time for attending the Muny Opera.

I watched people entering and quickly filling row after row of seats, and while waiting for the opening scene of the musical *42nd Street* I wondered just how many people—how many million people over the years—had viewed performances at St. Louis's renowned municipal opera.

Leafting through my program, I soon learned that 42 million persons have seen Muny performances with such stars as Bob Hope, Vincent Price, Ethel Merman, Red Skelton, Pearl Bailey, Angela Lansbury, and Carol Channing, to name a few. And there's a long line of Muny performers who had their start here and have gone on to Broadway and greater success.

The Muny, which holds a special place in the hearts of all St. Louisans, was built in 1917 for several performances of *Aida* produced by Guy Golterman for an Ad Club convention. Encouraged by the success of this endeavor, a Municipal Theater Association was formed. By 1919 the first of regular weekly shows began.

On opening night of the second show, *Bohemian Girl,* a violent rainstorm swept sets, properties, and musical instruments down the nearby River Des Peres. According to Muny history, only the fortitude of civic leaders saved the Muny. Henry Kiel (mayor) led a group that raised enough money from local firms to offset more than 70 percent of the loss. The next season was a success, and the rest, as they say, is history.

The Muny, pioneer of all outdoor summer theaters, is the nation's most famous one. It is the largest (twelve thousand seats) devoted to musical plays. It has a huge stage between two large oak trees, and its revolving central platform permits a scene change in a matter of minutes.

Next week, along with several other COTG residents, I plan to see *Singing in the Rain.*

June 22, 1986

The relatively new, young aide asked if I'd heard the announcement that dinner would be delayed one hour. I hadn't but wondered what the hang-up was. The aide said, "Suppose there was another water fight in the kitchen like last time?"

That was news to me, but visualizing the scene, I chuckled and went on my way. Now, I wonder what Mrs. Bono said if she knew and if that was the cause of the delay. I doubt if she chuckled.

Lack of responsibility can be entertaining and fun, I thought.

June 23, 1986

A neighbor COTG resident stopped by my room this morning. Noticing three books on my bedside table, she asked what I was reading. I told her, *The Memoirs of Heinrich Schliemann,* by Leo Deuel, Edmond Taylor's *Fall of the Dynasties,* and *Samurai and Silk,* by Haru Matsukata Reischauer, the Japanese wife of Edwin O. Reischauer, former ambassador to Japan."

"I mean what are you reading?" she queried.

"All three," I answered.

She looked at me as though I had three heads and said, "You can't possibly read all three at once."

"No," I told her, "not all at once, but concurrently, over a short period of time."

I thought later that I hadn't explained my reading habit to her very well. Just as I don't eat ham and eggs or chocolate cake at every meal, I like variety in my reading, too.

I think my habit of always reading at least two books concurrently goes back to my school days, high school and college in particular. I liked the change of pace of going, say, from a geometry class to one in English lit or from ancient history to chemistry or geography to physics. I found it kept me on my toes and always interested in pursuing some subject or other.

Today, at seventy-eight, I still like to pursue various subjects. Rightly or wrongly, I think it keeps me mentally alert.

June 29, 1986

From all I read and hear about other nursing facilities, I doubt there are many, anywhere, that do as much for or offer as many activities for residents as COTG. Not only are we given a wide choice of field trips, such as being taken to the Muny, the symphony, et cetera, we are also given a wide choice of entertainment here at the nursing home.

Today, for example, there was a bridal fashion show in which wedding gowns belonging to residents and staff were modeled. From the expression on most faces, I'm sure many beautiful memories were relived here today. Following the show, which was emceed by Dolores Silies, activity director, a very large wedding cake was cut and served with champagne.

June 30, 1986

Before going to COTG's bridal fashion show yesterday, I watched the William F. Buckley "Celebrity Roast" (a repeat), which took place last February celebrating the twentieth anniversary of "Firing Line" and Buckley's hosting of that program. I enjoyed it again!

As usual, Mr. Buckley's attire reminded me of an unmade bed and his disarming smile seemed to turn every roast into something close to a plaudit. No wonder even those who disagree with him most violently can't help but like him, if not his conservative philosophy.

Sunday, July 6, 1986, late

I just turned my TV off. . . .

America wore her heart on her sleeve this weekend! And she wore it proudly for all the world to see! I don't believe any American who saw or heard even a small part of the Liberty weekend celebration could avoid saying, "Thank God I'm an American."

Millions, whether American or other freedom-loving people, must have been misty-eyed with emotion or at least found it difficult to swallow the lumps that welled up in their throat. Whether it was President Reagan rededicating the restored Lady, lighting the beckoning new torch, or watching the international flotilla of tall ships (from thirty countries) honoring America with their twenty-one-gun salutes, or just listening to the stirring music and heartwarming speeches of well-known and little-known people, it was an emotional weekend few Americans will ever forget. I know I won't.

The weekend lingers on!

I'm still thinking about some of the activities and scenes that were televised:

1. The swearing-in of new citizens.
2. The honoring of some of our naturalized citizens.
3. The beautiful musical tributes, such as the New York Phil-harmonic concert in Central Park, with Placido Domingo and Marilyn Horne as soloists.
4. The stirring star-studded finale held in Giant Stadium.

And these are but a few of the highlights.

I mentioned the honoring of some of our naturalized citizens. When I saw the white-haired gentleman who rose in answer to the name James Reston, it was difficult for me to reconcile him with Scotty, the jaunty golfing newsman I knew in Dayton. Of course, that was some time before he became the internationally known syndicated columnist of the *New York Times.*

After writing the above, I took from my bookcase *The Kingdom and the Power,* a book I had given to Morgan on our thirty-second wedding anniversary. Then it was the newly published story of the *New York Times,* authored by Gay Talese, a *Times* staffer. Because he had mentioned Reston in the book innumerable times, I asked Scotty if he'd inscribe the book with a word or two. He wrote:

To Wanda and Morgan
Happy Days
Happy Memories
James Reston
November 24, 1969

Note: Morgan's and my anniversary was November 26, but what's a couple of days when memories are so precious?

Now I wonder how many of my friends from those long ago days would recognize me today, bent out of shape as I am. Not many, I wager.

July 12, 1986

I recently reread Lewis H. Lapham's editorial "Imperial Masquerade" in the last issue of *Harper's*. On first reading I thought he sounded like a young man trying to be "cute" in an effort to attract the attention of the literati. I felt he could have punctured the complacency of the "plutocracy" without resorting to ridicule and sarcasm.

The second reading makes me think that what he wrote probably pricked my own pomposity. That is, if his "pomposity" and "plutocracy" mean free enterprise, free trade, judicial restraint, and admiration for those Americans who use their mind and hands for work and not reaching for handouts, then I'm guilty.

Morgan and I worked hard all our lives. By careful management and investment. I'm now able to maintain myself in comfortable dignity. I never want to be a physical or financial burden to anyone—least of all Uncle Sam.

I hope that independent attitude doesn't make me one of Mr. Lapham's "plutocrats."

July 16, 1986

Periodically I remind myself of the many blessings that have come my way. *Life has been very good to me,* I thought last evening as I sat in air-conditioned comfort watching and listening to Richard Hayman and the St. Louis Symphony Pops.

Perhaps it was the nostalgic music (*Songs from the Silver Screen*), but in no time I was ruminating and reminiscing about some of those blessings:

1. As long as I can remember, I loved and respected my parents. They were responsible for my happy childhood and girlhood. They encouraged my education and instilled in me my love of books and music.
2. I married happily and well and was able to combine a successful career with a very happy marriage.
3. I was lucky in that the severe stroke I had didn't affect my mind (or so I'm told). My left side is completely paralyzed, but I've learned to manage quite well and all in all I live an orderly, normal life.
4. And how fortunate I am that I chose to live in a nursing home whose director and staff are caring and where activities such

as the Symphony Pops and Muny are regularly offered. That doesn't include the daily entertainment, games, small combos, singers, movies, art or cooking classes, et cetera, that are on the activity agenda. Last week I attended the Pops when Patti Page was the vocalist. The week before, sixteen residents (seven of us in wheelchairs), nineteen family members, and nine staff members boarded the *President* for luncheon and a three-hour cruise on the Mississippi.

5. And I haven't even mentioned my wonderful friends, who haven't forgotten me.

July 19, 1986

Just when you've decided life isn't easy, you begin to realize that nothing in life is ever too hard. That paraphrase, along with "Dying is an art. Baloney. It's living that is an art," are bits of sophistry from that delightful off-Broadway show *Taking My Turn.*

I watched the PBS repeat of it last evening and chuckled through it again.

Like the characters in the play, I too wonder whatever happened to "Please" and Thank you?" I'd like to add a few wonderings of my own such as:

1. Being on time. (It's a courtesy to the other person and only good manners.)
2. Saying, "I'm sorry."
3. Returning borrowed books.
4. Clean-shaven men. The current crop of bewhiskered males reminds me of push brooms. Upend them, use their legs as a handle, and push. Their whiskers could push-broom a floor in no time.

July 20, 1986

The news that May Company is buying out ADG (Associated Dry Goods) has left me with mixed feelings (the same stirred-up emotions I had when ADG bought old Stix, Baer and Fuller).

Financially, I'll benefit, as I've never sold any of my ADG stock. Sentimentally, I don't like to see it happen, as it's another step in the progression of chains and conglomerates taking over the fine old department stores of the country.

Having worked for a once-family-owned store and knowing both

ADG and May Company are good organizations, I still can't help but feel as Marjorie Rosenberg did when she wrote in the *American Scholar* Magazine.

> Like divine providence in an earlier age, economic forces now constitute the ultimate explanation for the way things are. Thus, when economic causes are identified for the indignities we suffer, inquiry ceases and we give ourselves up to resignation. So it has been with the passing of the Golden Age of the department store—a period that spanned some seventy years from the 1880's to the 1950's. The names of the founding families of these fine stores across the country have been retained as the chains and conglomerates that bought them out in the fifties and sixties steadily lower the quality of their goods and services and blaspheme their principles of doing business. But the transition from family to corporate ownership is neither a sufficient cause nor a justification for the evil it has brought.

I've always considered it a privilege that I had the opportunity to work for Stix, Baer and Fuller when it was family-owned and employees were made to feel they were part of the family.

Values of the heart still mean more to me than values of or in the pocketbook. In today's economy, I suppose that's a stupid thing for me to say, but I'm put together with those bolts and screws and I in no way regret it.

July 25, 1986

Stopping me as I left the dining room today, one of COTG's newer residents asked if I had gone to "that disgraceful show the other evening." Before I could reply she continued impatiently, "You know, that caged folly thing."

Realizing she meant *La Cage aux Folles,* which I and several other residents had attended at the Muny, I said, "Yes. I thought the musical extremely well done."

Noting the disapproving look on her face and not wishing to get into any discussion on morality I amplified my comment by saying, "A bit risqué perhaps but— . . ." I got no farther, as she interrupted with, "What in the world did you find good about it?"

I explained that I thought the choreography was outstanding, the costumes beautiful, and the sets quite effective. She gave an audible snort and with a distinct "Humph" strode off, leaving me with the feeling I must be headed straight for Dante's Hell.

Later, mulling over that resident's reaction and obvious disapproval, I thought that homo- and transsexuality are facts of life and disapproval won't alter that fact. However, *how* that fact is handled would justify society's approval or disapproval—not the *fact* that can't be changed.

July 26, 1986

Along with several other COTG residents, I enjoyed a delightful few hours last evening when we watched and listened to that likable, very talented "ham," Richard Hayman, lead the St. Louis Symphony Pops down "Memory Lane."

The Cosmopolitan Singers and two versatile vocalists, Katherine Terrell, soprano, and Lewis Dale von Schlanbusch, baritone, were features of a nostalgic program of Lerner and Loewe hits.

Songs from *Gigi, Camelot, Paint Your Wagon, Brigadoon,* and *My Fair Lady* left an enthusiastic audience applauding all through the memorable program.

As usual, after such an evening of songs, I went to bed humming scattered bits from "If Ever I Would Leave You," "I Remember It Well," "Thank Heaven for Little Girls," "Heather on the Hill," "I Could Have Danced All Night," and on and on. . . .

Yes, I finally and happily went to sleep.

August 4, 1986

Words and their connotations intrigue me.

In glancing at the paper in front of me, the word "integrity" caught my eye. I don't know how the word was used, as I haven't read the article as yet, but to me there is no more descriptive word for moral character than *integrity.*

As for the words *moral* and *character,* I think one could spend a few very interesting hours delving into the many ramifications of those two words.

I know I can spend an afternoon idly leafing through a dictionary—following up definition after definition. There's only one drawback. Having the use of only one hand and arm, I can't manage my large, comprehensive dictionary, and paperbacks, like the one I just dropped, last me no time at all. The pages come unglued and fall out, and I'm a blithering idiot by the time I locate the word I'm

seeking; I think I've called every bookstore in St. Louis trying to locat
a good, hardback *small* dictionary . . . one I can handle. I've writtei
to Barnes and Noble (supposedly the world's largest bookstore). S(
far I've had no luck.

Paul's Bookstore, a small, highly respected shop, just told m(
they have a small hardback dictionary, published in England, due
for delivery in October.

I left an order!

August 11, 1986

Mrs. Bono asked if I'd chair COTG's effort to support the Humane Society's benefit rummage sale. Feeling as I do about animals,
I'm ever so pleased to be of assistance.

In thinking about material and information for letters, posters,
et cetera, to encourage donations, I remembered the picture of two
Shar-Pei puppies that Carolyn Wilson had given me. They should
attract attention, I thought. They did!

Shar-Pei's are considered the world's rarest breed of dog. In the
1950s, there were only twelve in the world. When that was discovered, a worldwide plea went out to save the breed. In 1983 there
were 2,495 registered in the Shar-Pei Club of America. Prestigious
Neiman-Marcus, which prides itself on presenting the rare and beautiful, advertised Shar-Pei puppies at two thousand dollars each in
1983. The breed dates back to the Han dynasty in China (206 B.C.
to A.D. 220).

These lovable, wrinkle-skinned puppies (beauty, as we know,
is in the eyes of the beholder) are exceptionally intelligent and so
clean they often housebreak themselves within a period of a month.
Adult Shar-Peis grow into their oversize skin, which nature gave them
as a puppyhood defense mechanism.

The poster using the picture of the Shar-Peis is a hit, and COTG
residents and their families are enthusiastically backing the benefit.

August 15, 1986

I've been busy and happily doing what I can in organizing
COTG's effort to support the Humane Society's benefit rummage
sale. I'm currently going through my closets, chest drawers, and shoe
boxes to ferret out my unwanteds for the society's unwanteds . . . all
of which reminds me that I'd like to increase the bequest in my will
to the Humane Society.

I should review my will anyway to see if it still expresses my wishes and priorities. Aside from bequests to a few people, I'd like for whatever is left of my worldly goods to benefit the following and in the order listed:

1. Children
2. Education
3. Animals

Not that I'm anticipating my demise, but then who knows? I didn't expect my stroke either. Guess I'd better contact my attorney, Robert Meyer.

I do like things orderly and neat!

August 18, 1986

I wonder what I've been doing to deserve all the ten days I've been having lately. It can't *all* be due to music, although my attendance at the St. Louis Philharmonic Benefit and my several recent trips to hear the St. Louis Symphony Pops certainly played a large part in my enjoyment of daily living.

Too, I've again been traveling vicariously. Emily has taken time to tell me in detail about her most recent European trip. She spent time in London and the Cotswald area of England, then on to Scandinavia, where she cruised the fjords.

When she talked of Norway, I immediately envisioned Vikings, old ships, Edvard Grieg, clear blue water, and pine-covered mountains.

Sweden made me think of Carl Milles, the Millesgarden, and the old Stockholm Cathedral, which, if I remember correctly, celebrated its seven hundreth anniversary just a few years ago.

Her references to Finland occasioned thoughts of saunas, the Baltic, flower and fruit stalls, and of course Sibelius and his music.

Denmark brought back memories of captivating Copenhagen, the Little Mermaid, Georg Jensen, Kronberg Castle, Elsinore, and William Shakespeare's "Hamlet, Prince of Denmark."

Following her sojourn in Scandinavia, Emily spent a week in Russia visiting Leningrad and Moscow. Having never been in Russia, I was particularly interested in her cursory opinion of the people, museums, hotels, entertainment, and food.

Backtracking a bit, I'm now thinking of Norway's Thor Hyderdahl, *Kon Tiki* and *Ra II,* and the *Kon Tiki* museum in Oslo.

And how could I forget the fifteenth-century carved wooden sculpture of Saint George and the dragon in Sweden's Stockholm Cathedral.

I've had such fun mentally traveling the last few days.

August 24, 1986

Baudelaire and Proust expressed it, but the article "The Intimate Sense of Smell," by Boyd Gibbons, in *National Geographic's* September issue confirmed the *feelings* I've always experienced where smell is concerned.

I don't think I realized before that odors reach into all our emotional life, drawing from the deepest caves in our minds. Quoting from the article:

> Odors suggest, stimulate associations, evoke, frighten and arouse us but they seem to lie below conscious thought until someone like the poet Baudelaire parts the curtain.

> In bed her heavy resilient hair
> —living censer, like sachet—
> released its animal perfume,
> and from discarded underclothes
> still fervent with her sacred body's
> form, there rose a scent of fur.

I've felt but never expressed many of my feelings in the written word, certainly not as a Baudelaire or as a Proust in his *Remembrance of Things Past* when he said: "But when from a long-distant past nothing subsists, after the people are dead . . . taste and smell alone . . . remain poised a long time, like souls, remembering, waiting, hoping, amid the ruins of all the rest; and bear unflinchingly . . . the vast structure of recollection."

Apparently the sense of smell is at the heart of remembering and emotion. According to Dr. Michael Shipley, a neurobiologist at the University of Cincinnati College of Medicine: "The amount of brain tissue in man devoted to smell is very great. Although we don't seem to be very aware of smells, they have a very privileged access to those parts of the brain where we really live."

I have found that true. To this day, old as I am, the fragrant smoke from a good briar pipe conjures up pictures of Morgan. The smell of a wood-burning fireplace brings back memories of my parents' home and of Morgan's and my beloved Echo Valley.

It is certainly true, as Rudyard Kipling said: "Smells are surer than sounds or sights to make your heart-strings crack."

The Gibbons article is technical in many respects, but so well documented and so well written almost any layperson will enjoy reading it.

August 27, 1986

I learned today that the much talked about Baccarat Museum Collection sponsored by Neiman-Marcus will be shown in N-M's St. Louis store from September 29 through Christmas. The signed and numbered limited edition pieces will be offered for sale during that period at prices ranging from one thousand dollars to fifty-three hundred dollars. Each piece will be encased in a presentation box.

The Baccarat Company has been in existence for over two centuries. It has survived three revolutions and four invasions. Baccarat craftsmen have blown, cut, and polished by hand what is regarded by connoisseurs as the world's finest crystal.

As the story goes, about three years ago N-M representatives approached Baccarat with an ambitious idea. That idea was for Baccarat to create a special collection of decorative pieces, using design blueprints from the Baccarat archives. These re-created objects were once known only to the aristocracy.

The resulting collection spans one hundred years of Baccarat history from 1830 to 1930 and is said to offer a great variety of style and design—from the functional to the purely decorative. The collection has been carefully edited to twenty-three significant pieces. The thought behind the editing was to present those pieces representative of the evolution of design and creativity at Baccarat. These re-created pieces, in the originals, had been exhibited, had been especially commissioned by important personages, or had been especially difficult to make. Each has been made with the same painstaking workmanship as was taken with the originals. Some of the designs could only be made at the rate of two a month.

Since its inception in 1924, twenty-six Baccarat craftsmen have been awarded the coveted Meilleur-Ouvier de France—an award given out each year by the president of France to the country's finest craftsmen. No other French concern has won it so many times or has so many noted and active award-winning artisans working for it.

I am planning to see the exhibit.

August 31, 1986

From all I read and hear, it appears the tax reform bill will be signed, sealed, and delivered when the "congressional boys" return to Washington after Labor Day.

Our tax code certainly needs reforming, and from what little I know about such matters the new bill seems to me to be a great improvement over the complicated "Vhere iss my leff ear" rules taxpayers struggle with now. But then who am I to disagree with the economists who say there are too many flaws in the bill? Could it be those economists have become so accustomed to entitlement programs they really believe they're a fact of life?

I know the bill is far from perfect and may be flawed in many respects, but I have enough confidence in the American people to believe necessary adjustments will be made when needed.

I have almost always been on the side of management, feeling the entrepreneurs are the ones who take the risks in providing jobs for the rest of us as well as for themselves. The new bill as I understand it will put more tax burden on business (I think political compromise shows through here), but the same bill does away with tax shelters and deductions that have been enjoyed by too many for too long.

Perhaps the tax cut for most individuals will cause them to spend more and thus stimulate business. That, of course, remains to be seen.

All in all, I think it's a good bill and certainly an overdue step in the right direction. Only time will tell if it's revenue neutral. At any rate, I'm for giving it a try.

September 6, 1986

I doubt if I'll ever understand politics or politicians. Why, will somebody tell me, is Congress so insistent upon protectionism while at the same time state and municipal legislators vie with one another to see which ones can offer the best deals to Japanese companies to build automotive or electronics assembly plants in their localities?

We're not only confusing the Japanese with our conflicting talk and actions, we're opening the door for closer trade between the European community (Common Market) and the Japanese. All the while we continue to blame the "other guy" for problems that are essentially of our own making and for the trade deficit we're facing.

From what I read and hear from those whose opinions I respect, European and Asian manufacturers are already cutting back on purchases of raw materials, machine tools, and synthetic fibers, much of which until now has been purchased in the United States with dollars previously earned from U.S. purchases.

It seems to me foreign investment actually creates jobs in our country. According to some figures I read recently, in 1984 alone over eighty thousand jobs were created as a result of direct Japanese investment. I wish Congress would start worrying about the budgetary deficit instead of the trade deficit.

September 7, 1986

I'm still mulling over yesterday's journal entry. When will the government stop overspending? When will we fall back on the ingenuity and creativity for which this country is or was known? It's time we roll up our sleeves, start thinking and working, and stop bellyaching!

September 8, 1986

A very happy Grandparents' Day came to Clayton-on-the-Green yesterday. There were many kids, happy oldsters, and much merriment.

The carnival atmosphere permeated the building and grounds. There were pony rides, music, clowns, games, prizes, noise, and laughter . . . all preceded by a delicious luncheon for residents and their families.

Not having any grandchildren and knowing I was a mite too handicapped for a pony ride, I just sat and watched for a while, thoroughly enjoying the youngsters and the fun they were having.

When I returned to my room, I stretched out for a bit, trying to decide whether I wanted to read or take a nap. I was still trying to make up my mind when the Menhard family arrived: Chris, Donita, their adorable two-year-old Katie, three of Katie's little cousins, Jenny, Mindy, and Kristin, and Grandmother Shirley, Chris's mother. All had come to share Grandparents' Day with me. I was very touched.

Even today when I glance around my room and see the flowers they brought, I'm reminded of their thoughtfulness.

September 12, 1986

It was love at first sight! Her expressive dark eyes, curly hair, tiny feet and ankles made me think she was the most appealing little creature I'd ever seen. She was so dainty and petite I called her Trinket.

Trinket is my newly acquired teacup poodle, which Mrs. Bono is permitting me to keep in my room.

Helen and Joel Kurtz lent me their specially built doggie playpen that they had made for their poodles. The pen is large enough for a doggie bed, food and water dishes, and toys and with enough room left over for Trinket to romp and play, which she does by the hour.

That tiny little bit of fluff is making me the happiest oldster at COTG. Trinket is two months old, weighs one and a half pounds, and is so captivating she has won not only my heart but that of everyone else who has seen her.

September 18, 1986

Emily sent me the following bit of nostalgia. I relate to it because the rememberings are dated 1936—the year before I was married and an era that is fun and heartwarming to recall. I have no idea who the author is:

The Way We Were

We were before television. Before penicillin, the pill, polio shots, antibiotics and frisbees. Before frozen food, nylon, dacron, Xerox, Kinsey. We were before radar, fluorescent lights, credit cards and ballpoint pens. For us, time-sharing meant togetherness not computers; a chip meant a piece of wood; hardware meant hardware; and software wasn't even a word. In those days, bunnies were small rabbits and rabbits were not Volkswagens.

We were before Batman, Rudolph the Red-Nosed Reindeer and Snoopy. Before DDT and vitamin pills, vodka (in the United States) and the white wine craze, disposable diapers, jeeps and the Jefferson nickel. Before Scotch tape, M&Ms, the automatic shift and Lincoln Continentals.

When we were in college, pizzas, Cheerios, frozen orange juice, instant coffee and McDonalds were unheard of. We thought *fast food* was what you ate during Lent.

We were before FM radios, tape recorders, electric typewriters, word processors, Muzak, electronic music and disco dancing. We were before pantyhose and drip-dry clothes. Before ice makers and dishwashers, clothes dryers, freezers and electric blankets. Before men wore long hair and earrings and women wore tuxedos. We got married first and then lived together. How quaint can you be?

In our day, cigarette smoking was fashionable, grass was mowed, coke was something you drank and pot was something you cooked in.

In our time, there were five-and-ten-cent stores where you could buy things for five and ten cents. For just one nickel, you could ride the street car, make a phone call, buy a coke, or buy enough stamps to mail one letter and three postcards. You could buy a new Chevy coupe for $600, but who could afford that in 1936? Nobody. A pity, too, because gas was eleven cents a gallon.

We were before vending machines, jet planes, helicopters, and interstate highways. In 1936, "made in Japan" meant junk; and the term "making out" referred to how you did on an exam.

We were not before the difference between the sexes was discovered, but we were before sex changes. We just made do with what we had.

And so it was in 1936. . . .
This is "THE WAY WE WERE"—and
WE LOVED IT!!!!!

September 21, 1986

Yesterday one of the residents and I were discussing the attitudes and abilities, in general, of the young people of today. Using her own children as examples (two girls and a boy—all married), she wondered if it wasn't more difficult for young marrieds today to face up to adversity, even commonplace disappointments, then it was for young people of earlier generations.

I don't doubt but that today's young have been given more advantages, have known a higher standard of living, are better educated (I think that might be debatable), and are living in a society that too often expects help when the going gets rough.

As we talked, I was reminded of a letter from a young married woman written to Morgan and me several years ago. I still have the letter.

Her mother had been my assistant when I worked for the *Dayton Journal-Herald*, and her father was a reporter for the same newspaper. When the two married, I was her mother's matron of honor. The couple eventually moved to Chicago, where her father took over a responsible job with a large Midwestern organization. They had four lovely daughters. The letter to which I referred was written by the oldest girl.

I question if anyone of any age in any generation could have faced up to a heartbreaking tragedy with greater inner strength, poise, and dignity than is evidenced in the daughter's letter, which follows:

Monday, September 9, 1974

Dear Wanda and Morgan,

All our lives we heard about you from our parents, and because of that I wanted to write you at this time. I don't know how much you were in touch with them during later years, or how much you knew about their lives then. So I don't know exactly how to approach this letter. You may even know already what's happened. In any case, I hope you'll understand how hard it is for me to write about it, and forgive me for having to bring you this bad news. Their lives had turned into a trap, and my Dad couldn't see any way out. So on August 8th, he shot my Mom to death, and then killed himself.

Mom was an alcoholic—I also don't know if you already knew that. We don't know why, whether it stemmed from some dissatisfaction with her life, or whether it was just one of those things that catches you and won't let go. It seems to have become evident during my later years in college, but I was away from home so much that I only figured it out five or six years ago. Dad didn't want to talk to us about Mom; it seemed to him like a betrayal. Later on he did, of course, but even then not enough.

For years she was in and out of hospitals; she saw a psychiatrist, but would never cooperate with him. She couldn't admit to herself that she was an alcoholic; and she blamed Dad for everything: losing her job, being hospitalized, us knowing.

Early last summer Dad moved out and said he'd come home when she quit drinking. She wouldn't quit, but finally she got so sick that she had to ask to be dried out—that had never happened before. She promised not to drink, Dad came home, and we thought everything was going as well as could be expected.

But by then there was irreparable damage to her body and her brain. It was hell for Mom and Dad, and when he retired last fall he was home all the time, being hounded almost twenty-four hours a day. She still blamed him and she still wanted him to let her drink. This summer she began acting as if she were drinking—stumbling around, being almost inarticulate—but he knew she wasn't drinking. My sisters are nurses and they say that those symptoms can recur if you're in bad enough shape.

After her deterioration when she was alone last summer, he felt he couldn't leave her. And in a goodbye letter to us, found afterwards, he said he couldn't leave her to be a burden on us.

That's all I can think of to tell you except that they both died quickly. I had hoped all those years that his daughters could love him enough to compensate for what was going on at home. He had us through letters, phone calls, and visits with Georgia and her family, while the pain was always there at home. There were two Moms, and the one we loved first has been gone for years. It's Dad's death that seems so unnecessary.

I'm so sorry to bring you this news about your friends, my parents. I'd give years off my life if it weren't so. If I've left questions in your minds, please don't hesitate to write; I'd want to know everything if I were you, and for me the pain is in the loss, not the telling. Thanks so much for having been so dear to them.

September 25, 1986

Elvira called to me, "And how's our Trinket today?"
I answered, "Just fine, but she's such a little ham."
"Oh," Elvira replied, "I thought she was a poodle."

October 9, 1986

Today I read an article written by Thomas E. Witherspoon that referred to his father. I related to the article because it reminded me so much of my own father and the expression "Much obliged," which he frequently used. As I'd like to incorporate the attitude that expression evokes into my daily living, I'm going to copy excerpts from the Witherspoon article into this journal as a reminder.

Much Obliged!
by Thomas E. Witherspoon

The phrase "Much Obliged" is one that many people might consider archaic, but it is very meaningful to me. My father used it, and it meant much to him. "Thank you" was casual to him. "Much Obliged" was much more; it was a commitment.

When my father said "Thank you" it meant just that. He wanted the other person to know that he appreciated an act or gesture. When my father said "much obliged" he wanted the other person to know "I owe you and I will repay you in kind or something better."

In lean times during the 1930's and 1940's when someone gave my father some game or fish for our table, the response was always "Much Obliged." Then at the right time, in the right way, my father would repay the obligation. I remember one occasion when this happened. My father helped a neighbor pour cement for a sidewalk. After the task was completed, the neighbor opened his wallet and asked, "How much do I owe, Gene?" The response was instantaneous. "No charge. I'm obliged." The neighbor had given us fish several times in the preceding months. Both men understood the obligation and there was no further need to discuss the matter.

It worked both ways. I remember when a neighbor came to our home with a team of mules and a plow and turned over the soil in our garden. When he finished, my father asked the man what was owed. "No charge," he replied. "I'm obliged to you for all the tomatoes and potatoes and beans you put on our table last year."

Any dictionary will give a variety of meanings for the words oblige or obliged. The two primary meanings are: *to compel by moral, legal or physical force and to do a favor or kindness for one done.* The latter meaning was the one in action in my father's life. To compel was alien to his nature, just as it is to any person of high character.

Obliged is a beautiful word when there is no intent to compel, when the only things involved are fairness, honesty, sharing, loving and caring.

. . . In order to receive, one must give. In order to have much for which to be grateful, we must be a source of gratitude. We must think, say, and do the things that bring others to feel "Much Obliged" of us.

As I read the Witherspoon article I kept thinking, *I wish I had written that about my father.* He too deserved my gratitude for being the kind of person he was.

October 12, 1986

I've been so busy lately, watching and playing with Trinket, writing thank you notes for gifts she's received, that I've neglected making entries in this journal. It has been a very happy interlude, but it's time I started jotting down some of my thoughts other than those connected with one tiny dog.

October 13, 1986

The Reykjavik summit ended yesterday in disappointment . . . for everyone! Oldster that I am, having lived through many disappointments, both personal and general, I've learned that making an instant or even a quick analysis or appraisement of a situation can be counterproductive . . . even dangerous. I'll leave better minds than mine to interpret the nuances of the U.S.-Soviet relationship. I only feel (and don't ask me how or why) that discussions will continue between the two powers . . . perhaps not at a summit level at first, but discussions and progress will continue to be made. It doesn't make sense not to keep trying and I don't want any premature comment of mine, adverse or otherwise, to add to the speculation that is making the rounds.

I'm looking forward to hearing President Reagan's side of the story tonight. His perspective and perception are certainly worth hearing.

October 14, 1986

Last evening I listened to President Reagan and to all the comments, pro and con, regarding his actions at Reykjavik. I know I'll be called biased, but I can't see where he could do other than what he did, and I, for one, if this old lady's opinion means anything, applaud him for his patience and integrity . . . yes, and courage in standing firm. I believe history will so judge him.

October 15, 1986

While I have little confidence in humanity's common sense, I am less concerned about a nuclear holocaust than I am about the lack of morality and the increasing permissiveness that has and is insidiously invading our day-to-day living. What is more frightening to me is the public's cavalier acceptance of this deviation from Christian morality and ethics.

Barbara Tuchman, the Pulitzer Prize–winning historian, in a recent media interview said that people today can't or won't distinguish between right and wrong. When asked what she felt was most needed in the next century, she replied, ''Personal responsibility . . . responsibility for one's own behavior, actions and expenditures and not forever supposing society must forgive you because it's not your fault.'' Ms. Tuchman feels that the ''loss of the natural world that we live by: trees, water, the stripping of forests and damming rivers, the poisoning of the air, the loss of forests in the tropical world . . . all these things are raising real dangers and are already more with us than is the nuclear."

However, her main concern (as it is with many others I've learned) "is the deterioration of public morality." To back her concern she cites several examples, including "cheating in the stock market" and in politics, the sale of influence, and the corruption of elected officials.

October 17, 1986

My journal entries are certainly spasmodic, probably because my thoughts flit from one thing to another depending upon what I'm reading, hearing, or doing at the moment.

This evening I watched and listened to a roundtable discussion on business led by Louis Rukeyser. I was particularly impressed by John Heinz, senator from Pennsylvania. His comments regarding lawyers, while often hilarious, were as often true. As far as I know, this country is the only one where contingency fees are permitted. Rising insurance rates should remind us that we consumers pay in the end for a luxury that primarily benefits the lawyer.

October 18, 1986

Sally Unger, Mary Halloway, and Nell DeFord spent a few hours with me today. As always, it's so good being with and reminiscing with old friends. We're all about the same vintage and find we have many shared memories.

During our long rambling discussion and exchange of ideas, we wondered if John Heinz was thinking of entering the '88 presidential race. While we all wanted to know more about him, we all thought he had something to offer.

October 19, 1986

I gave my tickets to the special donors' concert to Carolyn W. While I always enjoy the symphony, I didn't feel quite up to a wheelchair trip today. There are times when I can't bring myself to inflicting the nuisance of a wheelchair upon my friends. Today was one of those times.

October 20, 1986

Today was a full, enjoyable, but very tiring day. My whirlpool bath this evening was very relaxing and very, very welcome.

I started out the day by voting this morning. (COTG arranges for us to vote by absentee ballot.) Following that, Carolyn took me to Dr. Williams's office, where X rays were taken and minor tendon surgery was performed on my left hand.

Carolyn and I then had luncheon at Neiman-Marcus, following which we visited the galleries to see the Baccarat exhibit. Because the exquisite crystal firefly left me admiring and asking questions, a gentleman in the department unlocked the showcase and took out the firefly for me to hold. I asked that he hold it, which he did. Then he suggested that I run my fingers over the crystal so that I could feel the delineation and detail. It was a beautiful experience.

Carolyn and I returned to my room late in the afternoon to be ecstatically greeted by Trinket. She gave a small plaintive cry when we opened the door that seemed to say, "Where have you been? I thought you had abandoned me!" Of course, I cuddled her in my arms, thinking, *How can anything so small give so much love and affection?*

October 22, 1986

Another full and enjoyable day. Mrs. Bono and staff loaded twenty-five of us, wheelchairs and all, into two COTG vans for a trip to Pere Marquette Park.

The drive along the river road was autumn—colorful and enlightening. The Mississippi was still high but gradually and obviously receding. No small craft were out, but barges and tows were slowly making their way upstream.

At Pere Marquette Lodge we were served a family-style chicken dinner complete with cole slaw, mashed potatoes, honest-to-goodness country-style cream gravy, corn, green beans, and homemade peach cobbler. It was delicious! Another long day, but oh so enjoyable.

At the dining table I sat next to Anna S——, a lovely ninety-three-year-old resident who was enjoying the outing as much as I. To her the trip brought back memories of the days when she visited nearby Alton. Her son, now seventy, was then thirteen and enrolled at Western Military Academy in Alton. She happily recalled her many visits and her son's pleasure in the school.

I was reminded of Morgan's and my boating days on the Mississippi and the many times we had anchored at Pere Marquette and had taken guests to the lodge for dinner.

Again my whirlpool was relaxing and very welcome. Six hours in a wheelchair tires my back, wearies my posterior, and prompts my paralyzed leg and foot to spasm. But the day was worth the aches and fatigue.

October 25, 1986

I just finished reading Christopher Buckley's *The Washington Mess.* I don't know when I last chuckled through a book. This "memoir" is delightful and should stop or at least slow down the flood of "memoirs" that have come from the White House during the last several years.

My first reaction was that the manuscript should have been "neutralized" before publication. Upon second thought, however, I wondered if unadulterated satire should be "neutralized"—especially if that satire combines slapstick lunacy with truth and reality so artfully it makes sense. No, it shouldn't be "neutralized," I decided. I hope Ken Wilde agrees, as I plan to give the book to him for his birthday.

November 2, 196

I doubt if anyone who isn't handicapped and/or physically hurting can or could understand the apprehension most of us nursing home oldsters have when a trainee aide attempts to transfer or handle us. I try to be tolerant when I'm unwittingly pulled, poked, or yanked.

I understand new aides must be trained. But why so many so often? What is wrong that so many of the new aides don't stay? Is the work too hard or too disagreeable? Are we residents too demanding or too difficult? Is the pay too low? A private duty nurse for part of the day is the answer for some of us. But having that kind of care on all shifts would require 'round the clock private duties. That expense added to what we already pay for nursing home care makes that kind of attention prohibitive. Maybe someone will come up with the solution.

I personally feel higher requirements to weed out or screen applicants is the first step. Higher pay for those hired and, if necessary, higher rent for residents might be the next step. I'd be willing to go along with almost anything or give up some other service to correct or at least slow up this almost constant "changing of the guard."

November 5, 1986

The vote is in and counted. The Democrats have taken over control of both the House and the Senate. Yes, I'm disappointed! Disappointed because I believe so strongly in the basic philosophy of the Republican party. I also believe and have faith in the democratic process and the will of the people. But knowing that will often vacillates and changes with the mood and situation of the moment, I can only hope liberalism doesn't make too many inroads into the philosophy of free trade, the right and *responsibility* of the individual to make his own way and shape the direction of his life, and judicial restraint.

Handout programs, except in the case of the really needy, to me are a disgrace and diminish the dignity of man.

November 9, 1986

I don't know why I am so amazed at Sam Donaldson's sanctimonious attitude when it benefits his political bent or panel discussion image. He's often smug and more often abrasive, and he usually annoys me. George Will, his panel companion, is politically biased, too, but somehow his comments and questions are more adroit, smoother, less strident and irritating—at least to me.

Could it be I'm annoyingly biased, too? Probably! Even so, I know I'll go on listening and being irritated by the shouting McLaughlins and the smug Donaldsons. It serves me right—but the different viewpoints give me something to think about.

I've been known to change my opinion.

November 16, 1986

For the past several days, I've found it difficult to locate or to even listen to the weathercast for trying to sort out and identify the following names and terms spewed out by the media: Jihad, Hashemi, I.L.M., McFarland, moderates, Hizbullah, Poindexter, holy war, Khomheini, Jacobsen, Party of God, hostages, extremists, and on and on ad infinitum.

Some say Reagan's credibility is on the line. If that is so, then

I don't know enough to be pessimistic about the outcome of his initiative in Iran. Until it's proved otherwise, I'll continue to accept him as a man of integrity trying to solve our problems by placing them into global focus. (I believe it was Norman Cousins who recently said man should start seeing and solving our problems in global terms.)

When the flak settles, perhaps more people will view President Reagan's efforts in the light of trying to help stabilize the volatile Middle East. Many people feel declining military fortunes combined with a very apparent succession crisis and worsening economy could or should, with encouragement, strengthen the position of the more moderate elements in Teheran.

I personally think Mr. Reagan sincerely believes a victory by Teheran in its long war of attrition with Iraq could open the door for an aggressive campaign by Teheran to sabotage and probably topple the moderate Arab governments in the Middle East. If his efforts failed in some areas. I believe his broad overall plan was good and justified.

I don't pretend to know much about foreign policy, politicians, and least of all about people like abrasive Sam Donaldson and smug Robert Byrd. Their "holier than thou" attitudes about the Iranian situation make me "madder'n hell." I seldom resort to such unlady-like language, but I do feel like doing so now.

November 19, 1986

Last evening, seven residents and three COTG staff members attended the opening St. Louis performance of *Cats*—that much talked about sell-out musical.

I knew the text was based upon the poems of T.S. Eliot primarily in *Old Possum's Book of Practical Cats*, but as it had been so many years since I had read Eliot and as I found it difficult to follow the lines of the poetry, I was left to make my own interpretation as the musical progressed.

I thought the staging, lighting, and costumes were dramatic, even spectacular, and I loved the miming and symbolic choreography. Too, not only Eliot's poetry hopped, skipped, and jumped through my mind, I was reminded of the efforts of other writers. The soft shoe choreography kept calling to mind Carl Sandberg's words about the fog creeping in on "little cat feet." Too, I kept thinking of another allegory, Christopher Morley's "Where the Blue Begins."

And, of all things, some of the tableaux (where "arms" or paws were raised in supplication) made me recall some of the steel engravings in Dante's *Inferno*, a large book in my family's library.

Cats will keep me occupied for quite a few hours as I've just asked the library for the *Collected Poems of T. S. Eliot*.

Back in my college days, when I was doing most of my serious reading of poetry, I wasn't too impressed with Eliot. (I probably thought him too avant garde then.) I do remember that he was born in St. Louis, lived in the East, and finally settled in England, where he became a British subject. When he affected an English accent, I recall thinking that was a little too much.

I don't question but that he was an outstanding poet, but whether he was as great as some people thought I have my doubts.

November 25, 1986

The flak over Reagan and Iran hasn't subsided, and it appears on the part of some Democrats that they're moving in for the kill. Some of the accusations and Comments remind me of a cartoon that came out during the confirmation proceedings of Chief Justice Renquist. The cartoon showed a pious-looking Senator Kennedy saying, "Quite frankly, Justice Renquist, I don't believe a man with your past history is fit for such a high position."

November 26, 1986

November 26, 1986 . . . a bittersweet day. Forty-nine years ago today Morgan and I were married. . . . He's as dear to me as he was on that long ago November day when we exchanged our vows of love and commitment.

Were we together now, I have no doubt but that we'd reaffirm that commitment to each other as we did each year on November 26.

I spent the morning in the office of Dr. Craig Aubuchon, the orthopedic surgeon who will assist my orthopedist, Dr. Joseph Williams, in operating on my foot.

I'm to go to the hospital on January 6 for more surgery on my foot and a bit more tendon cutting on my left hand. I hope more tendon snipping and splicing will relieve some of the muscle hurt (I don't know any other name for the pain) that I experience now. While I'm not looking forward to another stint in the hospital, I'll only be there a week this time around. It's the following six weeks in a cast that will make my daily living so awkward that casts a shadow now.

November 28, 1986

I seldom permit myself to impose "me and my wheelchair" upon my friends. Only on rare occasions have I visited in the home of a friend. I'm hesitant to do this because I feel that handling "me and my wheelchair" is a major production. When I have a nurse aide with me (which isn't always possible), I do not feel such an imposition. I made one of my few exceptions Thanksgiving Day.

When Chris Menhard (my former therapist) called to invite me to share Thanksgiving dinner with his family, I went through my usual reasons for not accepting. When I'd finished my litany, Chris chuckled and said if he and his wife (also a physical therapist) couldn't handle "me and my wheelchair," then we'd all better give up.

I accepted the invitation and had a perfectly wonderful time.

In retrospect, believing my friends are sincere when they say they wouldn't invite me if I were such a bother, I think my reluctance to accept their invitations is almost entirely due to my embarrassment in having to have assistance in the bathroom. As I have always been a very private person, this assistance has become the greatest embarrassment of my life.

December 3, 1986

Paraphrasing a well-known line, emphatically uttered by Alexander Wolcott (journalist, essayist, actor) in *The Man Who Came to Dinner,* I'd like to say, "I think I'll upchuck."

I'm figuratively sick to my stomach from listening to all the judgmental opinions being made regarding the "Iranian Affair."

I'm now more determined than ever to wait for the *facts* before altering my opinion of Ronald Reagan. For days I've listened to newscasts, panel discussions, the haranguing of politically disappointed senators, headline-seeking political aspirants, and the vitriolic comments like those made by liberal Moynihan and conservative Viguerie, et al. All of which makes me wonder what perversity, even streaks of cruelty, in people make good men, thinking men, take pleasure in the hurt or discomfort or another.

I'm reminded of a verse my father wrote many years ago. He

was an engineer, but he had a bit of philosopher in him, too, as the following will testify.

Words

Words are things—with sense and feeling;
With a definite form and shape;
Which cannot be changed in texture
After once their course is laid.

Words have souls like human beings—
With a purpose, object, aim,
Which can afloat on ethereal fancy,
Or can sink in densest main.

Words can lift to extravagant grandeur
The creative thoughts of man;
Or they can fetter creative thinkers
With a dint no charm can calm.

They can strike with sudden fury,
Like a stone or brick or flail;
Or they can soothe and calm the savage,
As no other source can wield.

Words can breath the breath of living
Into the low, transpiring soul:
Or they can blight the sublimest fancies
With their sting of death so bold.

Words have life like other beings
Which outlast the span of man.
They're the spirited, true expression
Of the inifinity of God's plan.

They are, perhaps, the most elusive
Of the qualities of grace:
Yet they can be the most constructive
Of all the finitudes of space.

Words can comfort and lend guidance
To the errant pilgrim here,
Or can sacrifice fondest friendships
Upon a barbed and cruel spear.

Words are truly Nature's marvel—
Truly greatest every way.
So be careful how you choose them,
How you use them every day.

December 4, 1986

Seven long years ago I moved to Clayton-on-the-Green Nursing Center. Since then I've called COTG home. As in any other day-to-day living, I've had my up days and my down days—days when I wanted to cry and did—days when only contentment and laughter filled the hours.

I've often thought "Between Laughter and Tears" could as well apply to my tenure here as it did to Lin Yutang's book.

This afternoon I'm planning to see Andy Williams's Christmas show at the Fox. What a pleasant way to earmark my Seventh Anniversary at COTG.

December 5, 1986

And what a pleasant afternoon it was. Christmas songs and romantic ballads kept me remembering and reminiscing about happenings and people I wouldn't forget even if I could. It was a long, physically tiring day, though. Nine residents and three staff members left COTG at 1:30 P.M. and returned at 7:00 P.M. Five and a half hours in my wheelchair left me feeling more bent out of shape than usual. After a glass of milk and a sandwich, I was eager for a whirlpool bath and bed. My left side actually throbbed, but the afternoon was and is worth the discomfort.

In bed I kept trying to think when it was I first heard Andy Williams. It had to be in the late forties or early fifties. I know he was singing with Kay Thomson, and I believe it was in the Rendezvous Room of the Plaza on one of my early trips to New York as a fashion jewelry buyer.

Still reflecting and trying to go to sleep, I read the "Facts Sheet about the Fabulous Fox" that one of the aides gave me as we were leaving the theatre.

Following are some of the facts, most of which I didn't know 'til now:

Built by: William Fox.

Opened: January 31, 1929, with *Street Angel,* a silent movie with Fox Movietone accompaniment, featuring Janet Gaynor and Charles Farrell.

Original Cost: $6 million. It was one of the first theaters built for "talkies" with central air conditioning and passenger elevators.

Furnished by: Eve Leo (Mrs. William Fox), who spent seven hundred thousand dollars for furnishing and appointments.

Seating capacity: Originally 5,060. Currently 4,665.

Size: Second in size to New York's Roxy Theatre, which is no longer in existence. Today, as a full-time operating theater, it is second in size to New York's Radio City Music Hall.

Length of lobby: 90 feet.

Height of auditorium: 116 feet.

Chandelier: twelve feet in diameter, frame made of gilded pot metal and art glass; *weight:* two thousand pounds; 160 light bulbs totaling 11,620 watts; and a total of 2,264 pieces of stained or faceted glass.

Backstage: eight floors of dressing rooms; only five have been restored.

Private screening room: Located in the basement; originally used as a rehearsal hall.

Closing date: March 1978 with a motion picture.

Purchased by: Fox Associates, Inc., in June 1981.

Restoration: Cost to date: $3 million. Plus 4,487 seats were completely renovated, 7,300 yards of carpeting were woven in the original elephant pattern, plaster molds were re-created, art glass was duplicated, ceilings were vacuum cleaned, the mighty Wurlitzer organ was completely rebuilt, the chandelier was relamped, and the stage was completely re-equipped with state-of-the-art sound, lighting, and stage technology.

Reopened: September 7, 1982, with the musical *Barnum.*

December 9, 1986

I spent the better part of yesterday listening to the House hearings on the Iran-contra affair. George Schultz and Robert McFarland testified. Poindexter and North are scheduled for tomorrow, William Casey the next day.

I suppose by the time the hearings are completely over, there will be contradictions and inconsistencies. (Isn't that true of most human behavior?)

Until it's proven otherwise, I'll continue to believe the best in each man. If I am wrong, then I'm the one who has made the mistake. If I'm right, then I've strengthened my belief in the *basic* good of and in man.

December 11, 1986

There *is* magic in music! I not only thought but I felt that last evening as I listened to the St. Louis Pops. Richard Hayman conducted the St. Louis Symphony in a program of Christmas songs and hymns. In addition, the Cosmopolitan Singers were on the program.

This well-known and much appreciated singing group has been directed for more than thirty years by Helen Louise Graves, who died November 27 of this year. As a memorial to her, the Symphony Society has dedicated the 1986 Holiday Pops concerts to her.

I had gone into Powell Hall not unhappy, but not exactly joyous either. It had taken longer than usual to load us into the van. It was cold, the wind was chill, and my coat seemed only to hold the cold closer to my body.

The evening ended with a songfest singalong in which the audience enthusiastically participated. The camaraderie was contagious and I noticed as "folks" filed from the auditorium there was warmth in their greetings and smiles on their faces. On my face, too!

As I was waiting in my wheelchair to be taken to the waiting van, four people (complete strangers) took the time to stop and wish me a "Merry Christmas." One couple even asked if there was anything they could do for me. My day ended on a ten plus note.

December 12, 1986

Today was another ten day. Gerry B. and Deeter Hedenkcamp stopped by to see me. Gerry brought a tin of homemade cookies for me and some puppy treats for Trinket. Deeter gave me a pocket radio, which I wanted and love, and not to slight Trinket, he played with her for quite some time.

I went to bed thinking how wonderfully kind and thoughtful most people are.

December 13, 1986

I've listened to everyone from billionaire Khashoggi, a Saudi, and the Iranian Ghorabanafar to Pat Buchanan, Moynihan, and "you name it," and I'm still withholding judgment until all the facts are in and some of the political flak subsides.

I hope before long the American people will arrive at a perspective (their own), not a perception created by rabble-rousing politicians. Has moderation gone out of our vocabulary and actions?

December 15, 1986

The annual COTG residents' Christmas party took place yesterday afternoon. The facility was wall-to-wall people, with residents, families, and friends. The buffet was extensive and elaborate. Marty Bronson entertained. Everything was beautifully planned and executed.

Santa Claus climaxed the afternoon when he arrived by helicopter and guests were taken to and from their cars by two old-fashioned horse-drawn carriages.

From the laughter and pleasantries exchanged, it was evident Mrs. Bono had scored another success. My guests, Carolyn Wilson, her mother Helen, and the Patton girls, Linda and Allison, assured me they had an enjoyable time. I know I did.

December 18, 1986

Often in the quiet of my room, I just sit, dream a bit, and let the outside world fade away. It is then my hurts, real and imagined, fade away, too, and I become a refugee from disappointment, frustration, and the weariness that stealthily steals into my body from time to time. Headlines and the turmoil of the world are far away, and I can and do commune with the inner me. On such occasions I feel refreshed and grateful that I'm alive and am able to laugh off the antics of our mixed-up world. Music and books take on a new dimension and deeper meaning, and friendships become dearer and more treasured.

December 27, 1986

The wonder and glory of Christmas has come—and continues to fill me with the warmth of love and the caring friendship that has surrounded me this yuletide.

I am more grateful than words can express.

December 31, 1986

It's New Year's Eve and I'm waiting for three of my fellow wheel-chair travelers to join me in a toast to the New Year—with a glass of champagne and some party goodies. I've invited Kay W——, a valiant lady who lost her husband while she was in the hospital recovering from the amputation of her right leg and right arm, Ruth A., who has been confined to a wheelchair with MS since she was thirty-seven years of age, and Mickie F——, another to-be-admired lady whose loss of sight and paralyzed legs were caused by MS. Louise M—— would have been my fourth guest, but she was taken to the hospital last evening, we hope for a short stay. She previously had undergone an operation for a blocked leg artery.

I had ordered a gardenia corsage for each of the ladies, and I've sent Louise's on to her at the hospital so that she'll know I'm thinking of her and wishing her well.

Personally, I'm looking forward to another pleasant evening of jovial conversation and happy reminiscences. I have found that those who have lost the most are more often than not the most inspiring.

January 1, 1987

To Morgan on his birthday:

There's a chance you wouldn't recognize me now, but somehow I think you would.

Presently the left side of my body is trapped within me, refusing to do or follow the dictates of my mind, but my brain still functions and thus my mind knows and remembers the love and happiness we knew and shared. That knowledge helps the impaired part of me adjust. "make do," and get on with my day-to-day living. As a result, I'm doing my best to live each day to its fullest. I'm as content as I can be without you.

I thought you'd like to know that.